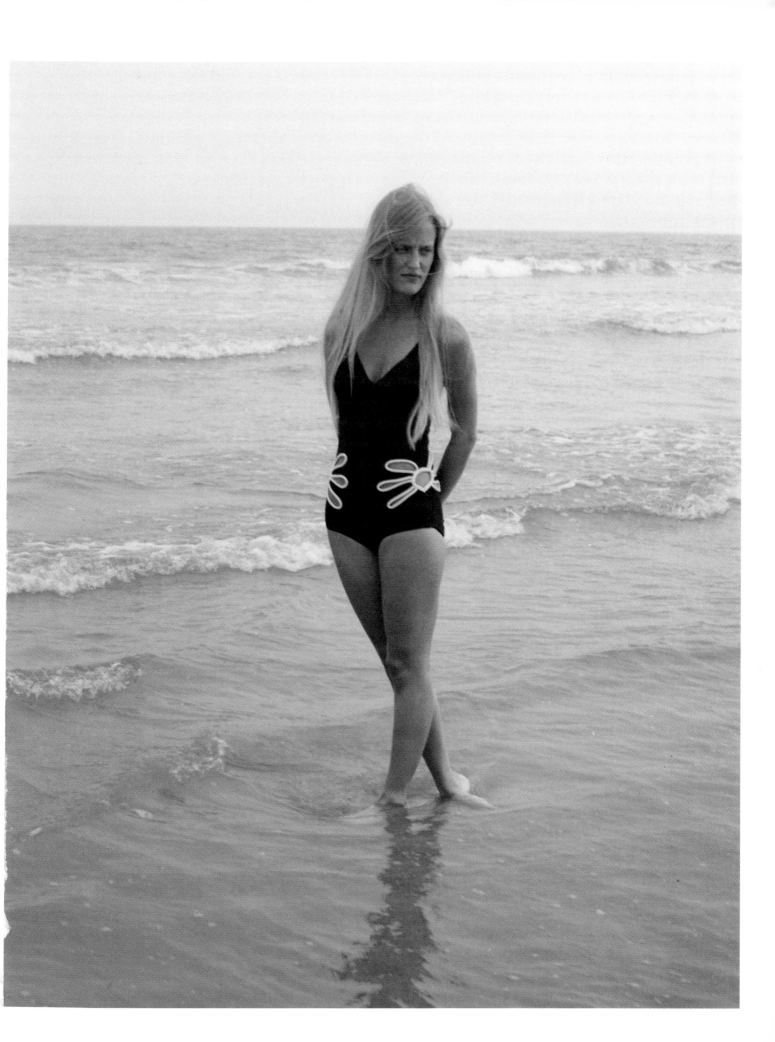

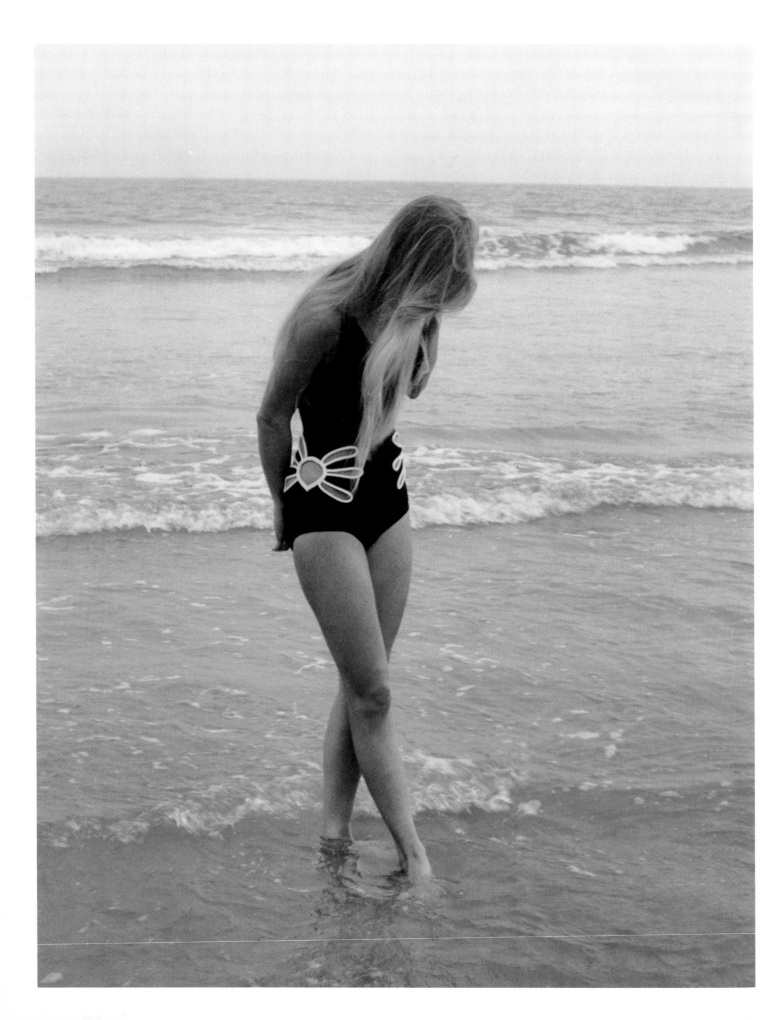

Vintage Style 1920 - 1960

Desire Smith

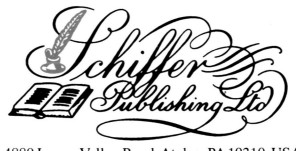

Schiffer Publishing Ltd

4880 Lower Valley Road, Atglen, PA 19310 USA

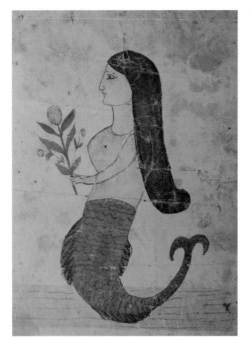

19th century mermaid, watercolor and ink on paper, found in Carlisle, Pennsylvania. *Courtesy of Bruce Smith.*

On the cover: Marcie Behanna, photographed by Desire Smith, wears a ca. 1950 halter style sequined sheath designed by Norman Norell, labeled Traina-Norell. Truly a "mermaid" gown, each sequin is applied flat, not overlapping, creating the visual effect of panne velvet. The model described this dress as the "most comfortable gown" she had ever worn!

Half title and title pages: Ca. 1950 black spandex bathing suit, decorated with white-edged floral cut-outs at the hip line; labeled Robby Len Fashions. An amazing bathing suit! *Modeled by Marcie Behanna.*

Library of Congress Cataloging-in-Publication Data

Smith, Desire.
    Vintage style, 1920-1960/Desire Smith.
        p.   cm.
    Includes bibliographical references and index.
    1. Costume--United States--History--20th century.
    2. Vintage clothing--United States. I. Title.
    GT615.S65   1997
    391'.00973'0904--dc21   97-19736
                                         CIP

Page layout by "Sue"

ISBN: 0-7643-0302-3
Printed in China
1 2 3 4

Published by Schiffer Publishing Ltd.
4880 Lower Valley Road
Atglen, PA 19310
Phone: (610) 593-1777; Fax: (610) 593-2002
E-mail: schifferbk@aol.com
Please write for a free catalog.
This book may be purchased from the publisher.
Please include $3.95 for shipping.
Try your bookstore first.

We are interested in hearing from authors with book ideas on related subjects.

This book is dedicated to the memories of my mother, Ruth Smith Munson, and my mother-in-law, Margaret Heath Smith.

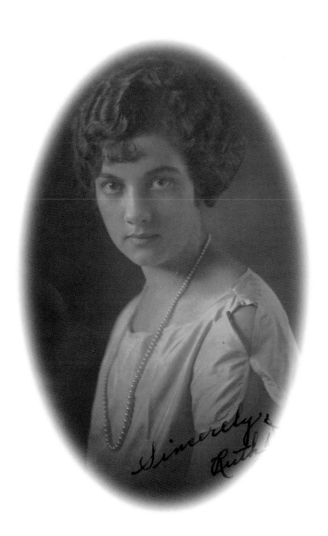

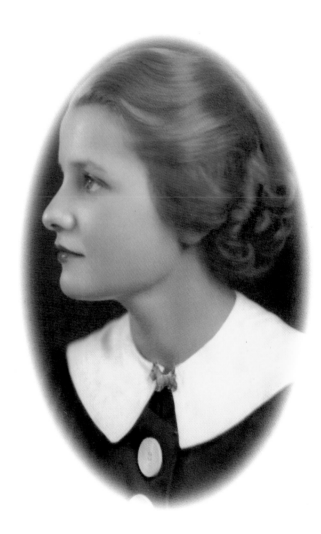

Preface

As a little girl, I was put down for my nap in my mother's bedroom. I would wait until the door was quietly closed, and, after lying still for what seemed to be a very long time, I would tiptoe from my mother's floral upholstered divan directly to her bureau, open the bottom drawer, and gaze at the array of beautiful sequined and beaded gowns she kept carefully folded

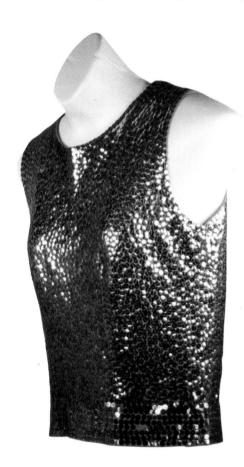

Ca. 1953 lilac silk jersey shell, decorated all over with lilac sequins, applied flat; attributed to NormanNorell.

there, gowns from her "flapper days." On particularly adventuresome afternoons, I would slip into my personal favorite, a lavender net, decorated all over with sequins. I would stand shimmering in sequins in front of her cheval mirror, tipped slightly toward me, so that I could see the bottom of the too-long dress piled up around my ankles. I don't believe I ever looked so beautiful as I did in 1948, at age four, in my mother's lavender dress.

I would like to say I have that dress today, or that I even know where it is, but I do not. What I do have is an intense interest in women's clothing and accessories, and a collection of the ones that appeal to me. Learning about fashion has been a life-long process, something of an obsession for me. I have always been aware of the ensemble effect of women's fashion. I believe every item a woman wears must be considered in relation to every other item she is wearing at that time.

Vintage Style is a fashion book about vintage clothing and accessories, mixing and matching, drawing attention to that one very special dress, handbag, pair of shoes, shawl, or hat. A number of photographs attempt to show that the back of a garment is stylistically as important as the front. Vintage clothing has become increasingly interesting, in recent years, to museum curators and preservationists, students of fashion and fashion designers, auction houses, dealers, collectors, costumers, reenactors, and those who may, or may not, fall into one of the above categories, but who clearly and unequivocally *live for fashion*.

Costume books generally focus on clothing from a particular period, giving an historical perspective. *Vintage Style* focuses on great style from diverse periods -- great style that is wearable today!

Desire Smith
April, 1997

Ca. 1953 Norman Norell sequined top

6

Contents

Acknowledgments

My sincere thanks to Peter and Nancy Schiffer for publishing my book, and special thanks to Nancy for your inspiration and help as my editor. Thanks to Sue Taylor, also at Schiffer, for your inspirational work as the layout artist for the book. Special thanks to cover model, Marcie Behanna, the "mermaid," for giving life to so many of the vintage pieces, and also to model Kim Hemingway for your beautiful presence in the book. Thanks to Douglas, Lois, and Emily Fischer for providing your lovely garden as a setting for some of the photographs--and Lois, thank you for permitting me to photograph several dresses from your personal collection for the book.

Thanks to my friends in the vintage clothing field for permitting me to photograph items from your personal collections or shops: Roslyn Herman (*Antiques and Celebrity Items*, Kew Gardens, New York), Lisa Miroslaw and Kevin Gallagher (*Decades*, Manayunk, Philadelphia, Pennsylvania), Karen Augusta (*Antique Lace and Textiles*, North Westminster, Vermont), Kelly Whalin (*Wear It Again Sam*, Manayunk, Philadelphia, Pennsylvania), Janet Milburn (*Somewhere In Time*, Lambertville, New Jersey), Stephen W. Sharpe and Karen L. Russell (*Past Tense*, The Power House, Collegeville, Pennsylvania), Matthew Smith (*Polyester Palace*, Antiques Marketplace, Manayunk, Philadelphia, Pennsylvania). Sincere thanks to Mark Walsh (Yonkers, New York) for providing images of the exceptional couture pieces from your collection, and Kelly Wright for the excellent photographs of Mark Walsh's pieces. You made a great contribution to the book!

And at Nesbitt College of Design Arts, Drexel University, thanks to Renee Chase (Department Head, Fashion Design) and Bella Veksler (Curator of the *Drexel Historic Costume Collection*) for permitting me to photograph items from the *Collection*; and thank you, Bella, for taking time from your busy schedule to discuss Nan Duskin with me and for your patience with my many questions about fashion history. Thanks to my nephew, antiques dealer David Sterner, for breaking your routine at auctions to buy a few vintage pieces for me to photograph for the book. Thanks to designer Louise Stewart for the enlightening interview.

Thanks to my friends Barbara Consorto and Angela Grimes for your computer expertise and your patience with a slow learner! Thanks to my friend and former art teacher, Donna Sigler, for "ferreting" out some great stuff, and to Gemma Pomilio for permitting me to photograph your wonderful red pocketbook. And to my many friends in the vintage field who have given and sold me items over the years, thank you. To Linda Becker and Donna Moyer (affectionately known to local auction goers as the "doily sisters"), thank you for the *Seventy-fifth Anniversary Issue of Hats*. To Larry Arrigale (Manager of *The Porch Cellar Antiques Market*, Chestnut Hill, Philadelphia, Pennsylvania), thank you for *The Wanamaker Diary, 1933*. The advertising was enlightening!

And finally, thanks to my family--my son Matthew, for your "eye for fashion" that has found some great pieces for me; my son Michael, for your willingness to carry far too many things upstairs; and my husband, Bruce, for being a patient, albeit harsh, critic--*sine qua non*.

Gold metallic threads woven on yellow/green crepe fabric

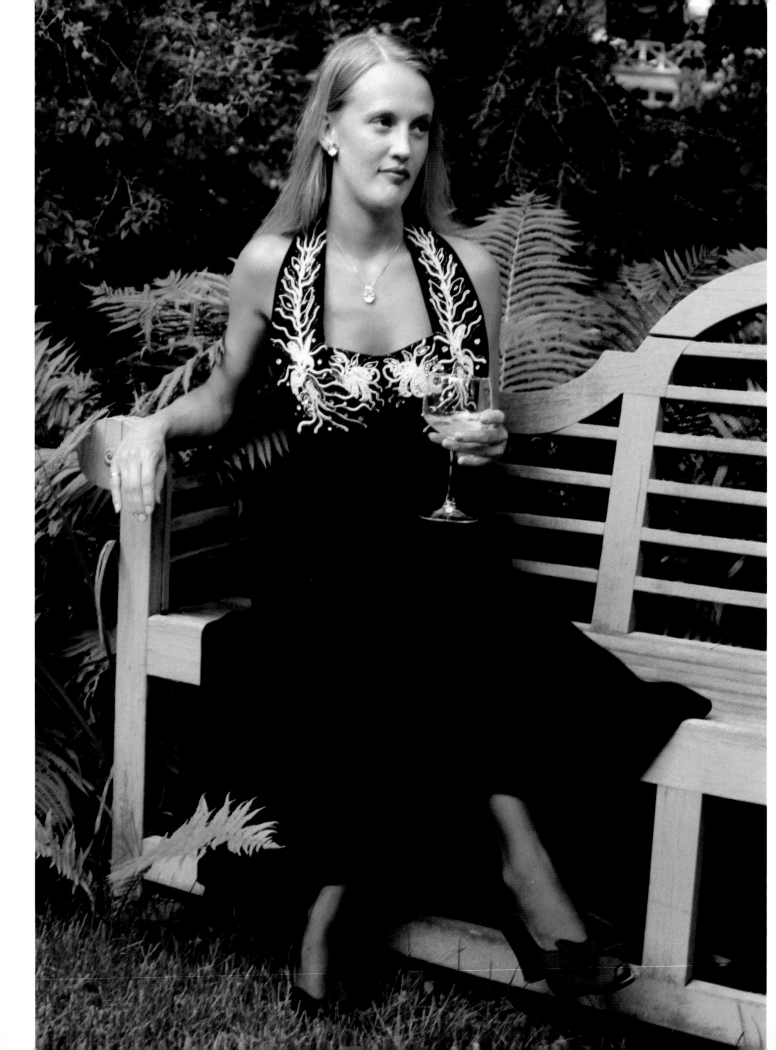

Chapter 1

Decades of Fashion

1920s

This is the era of F. Scott Fitzgerald and *The Great Gatsby*! Hats without exception are worn level, crowns ungracefully heavy and slipped deep over forehead and bobbed hair. Fashion critics of the day described the cloche as the "pot-shaped" hat; its variations "one more unflattering than the other." The chemise dress, with its fringes, sashes, and bead work is knee-length and somewhat shapeless. The practical limitation of the 1920s decorated chemise style, is that the heavy bead work from the bodice down, tends to cause the delicate shoulder straps to deteriorate.

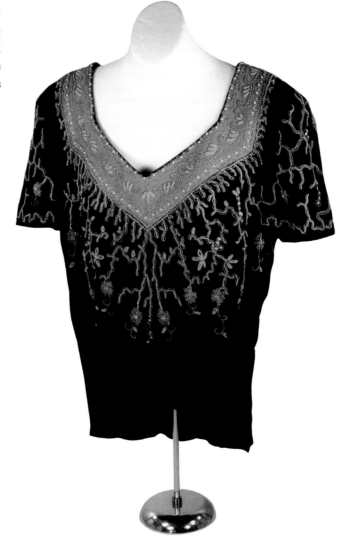

Ca. 1935 black and tangerine crepe blouse, decorated front and back with turquoise and coral beads, round, clear glass beads, and pearls. A striking piece!

Ca. 1950 black linen halter-style dress; bodice and straps elaborately decorated with soutache and rhinestones; attributed to Eisenberg Originals. Worn with signed Eisenberg pear shaped pendant, and matching earrings, set in sterling silver. *Modeled by Marcie Behanna.*

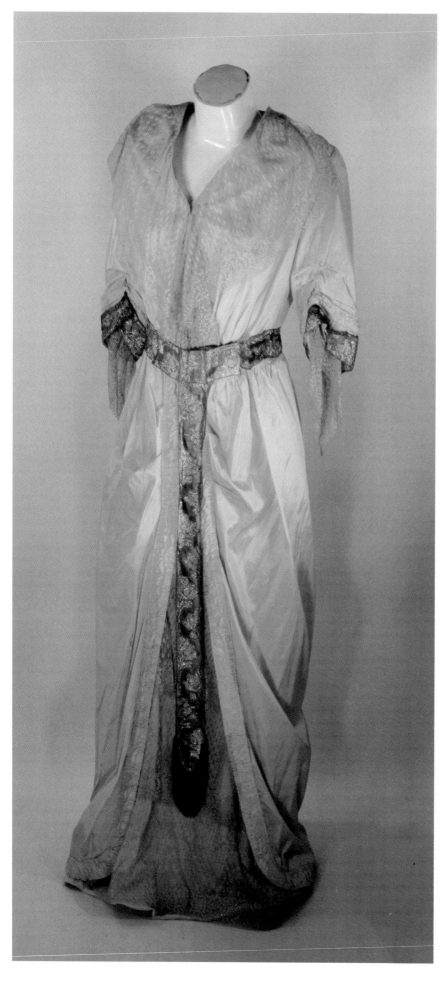

Ca. 1920 ivory silk gown, draped skirt; handmade silver metallic lace sash and trim at sleeves; attributed to Madeleine Vionnet; showing classical drapery, wide-open neckline, faggoted seams, Art Deco embroidery, suppression of hooks and eyes, and flawless sewing; labeled B. Altman & Company, Paris, New York.

1920s navy blue silk with metallic threads

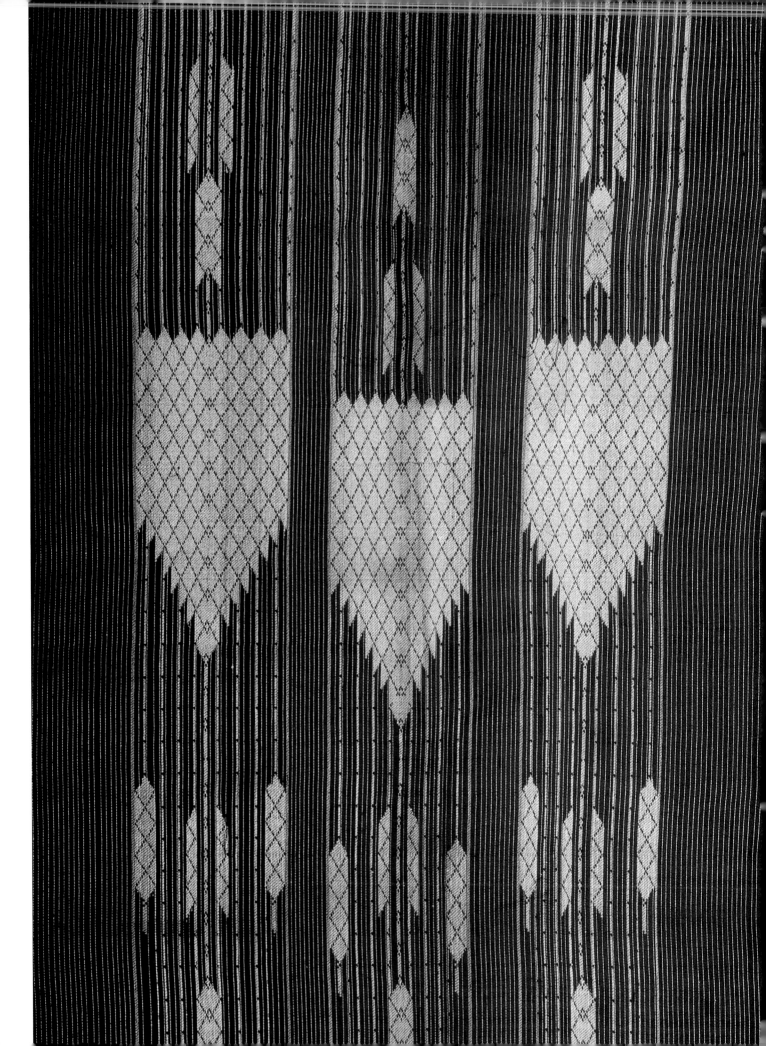

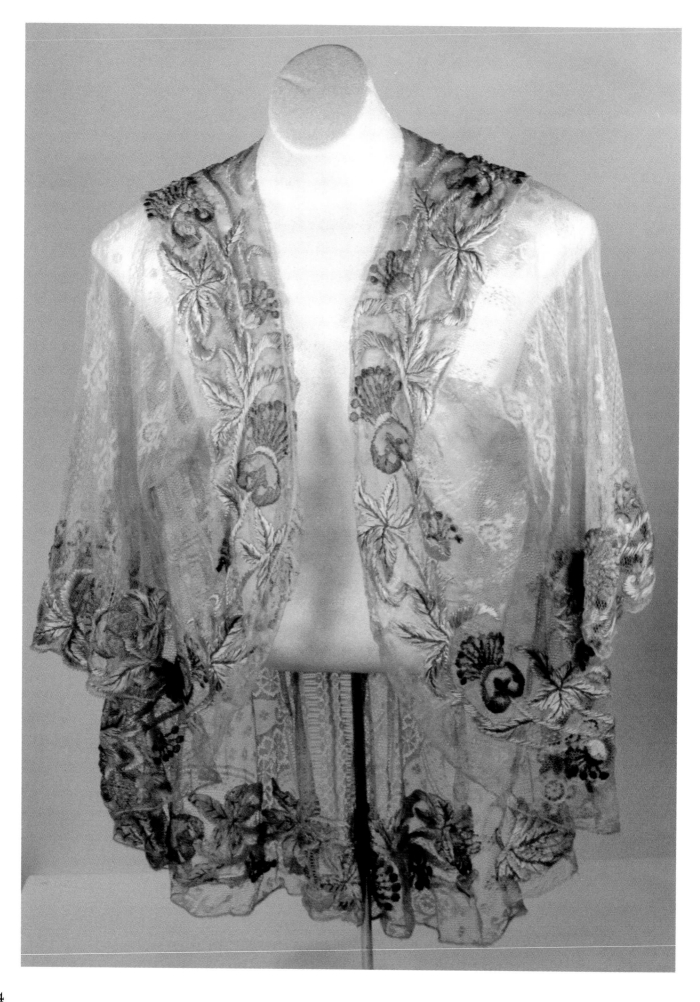

Ca. 1920 handmade lace bed jacket, elaborately embroidered with pink silk and metallic threads, in a floral design. Attributed to Callot Soeurs.

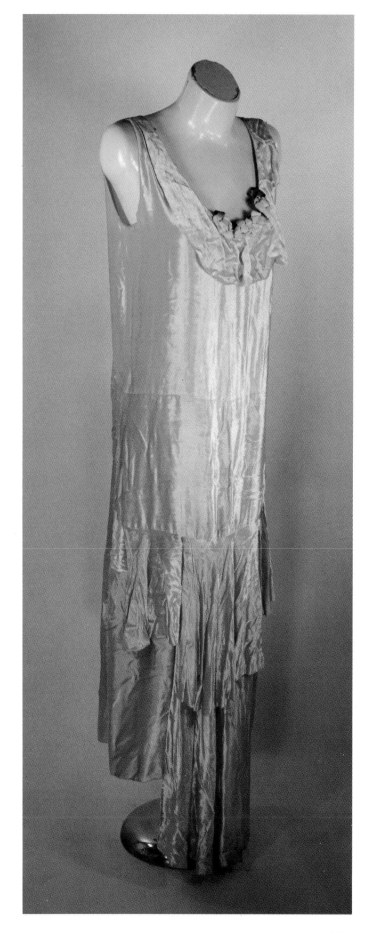

Ca. 1925 peach silk velvet gown, decorated with three cotton flowers at the neckline; uneven hemline. *Courtesy of Kelly Whalin.*

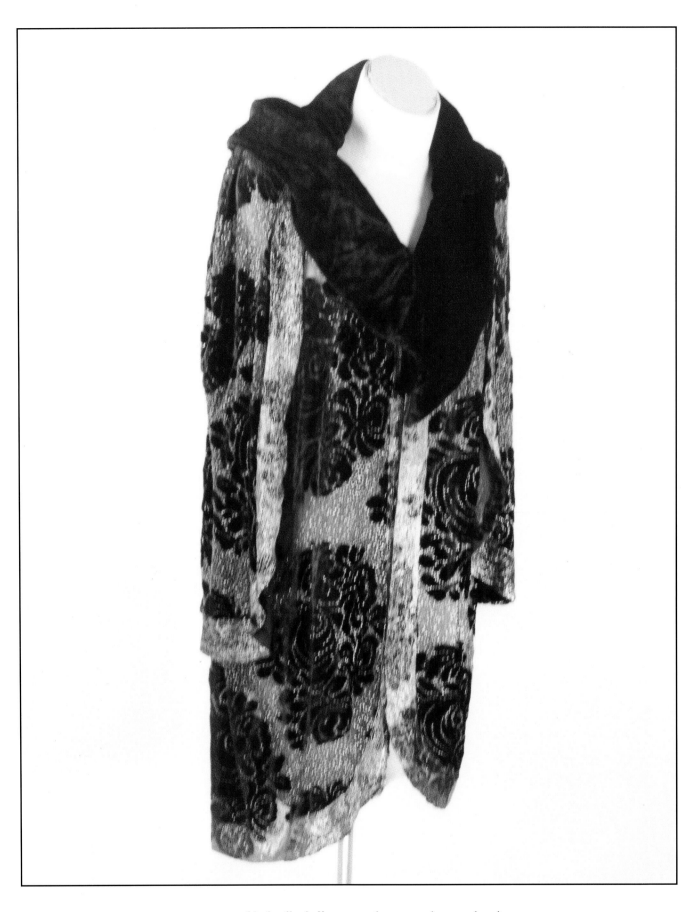

Ca. 1935 black silk chiffon, cut-velvet cape, decorated with round and bugle silver glass beads, in "swirls" between the large roses; black silk velvet collar; two layers. A truly incredible cape—a beautiful textile with intricate bead work, and exquisite design.

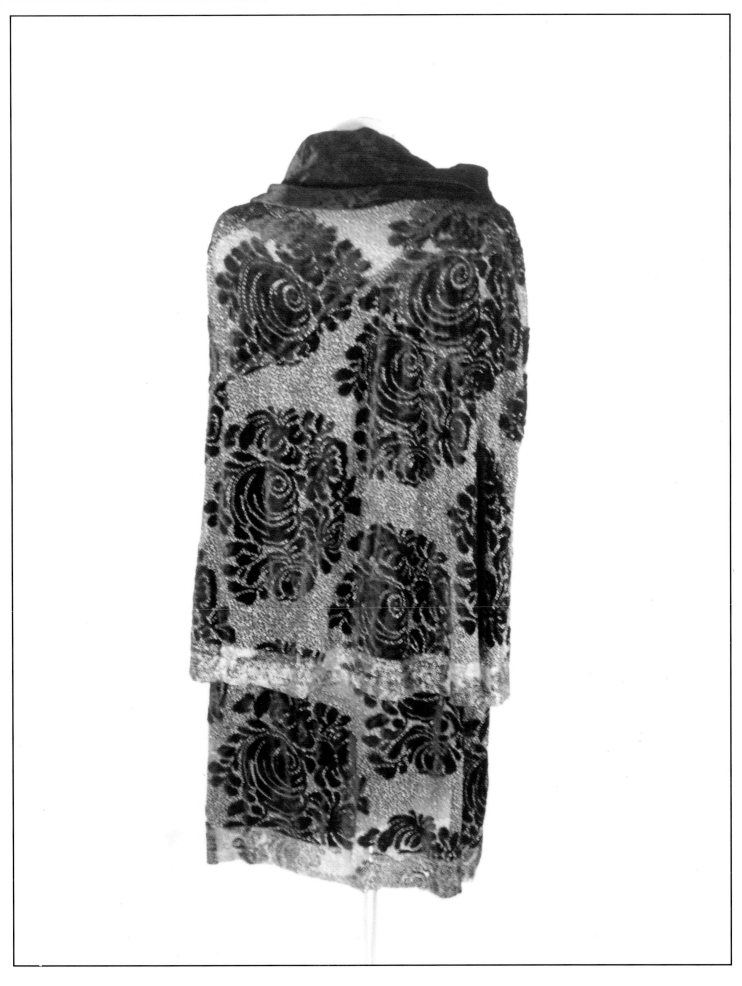

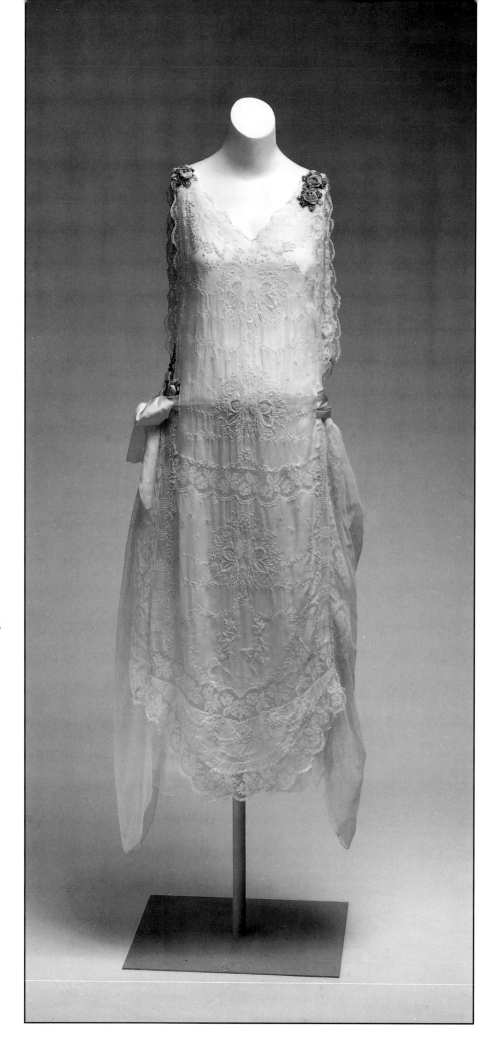

Ca. 1920 "lingerie" *robe de style*; white embroidered lawn with filet lace, cotton net, and silk ribbon rosettes; labeled Boué Soeurs. A fantasy of lace! *Courtesy of Mark Walsh.*

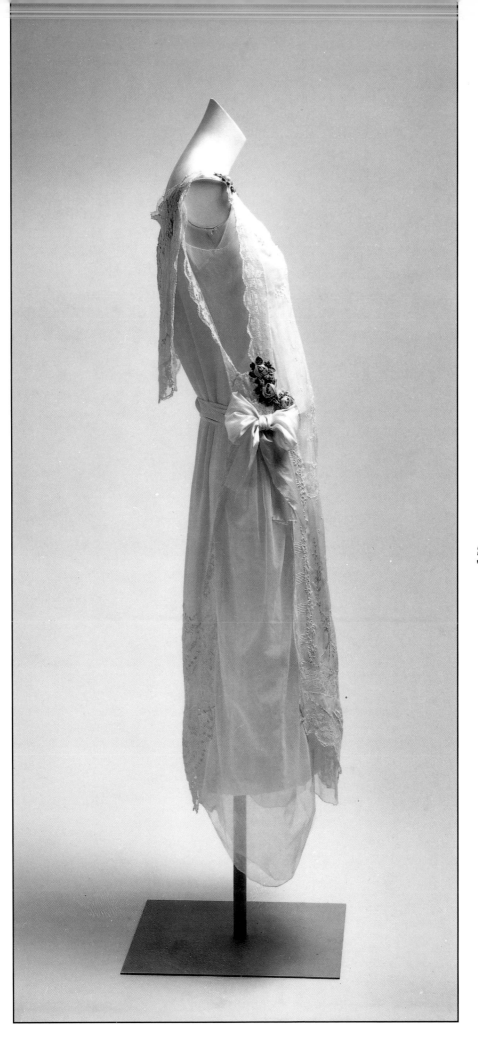

Side view of ca. 1920
"lingerie" *robe de style*.

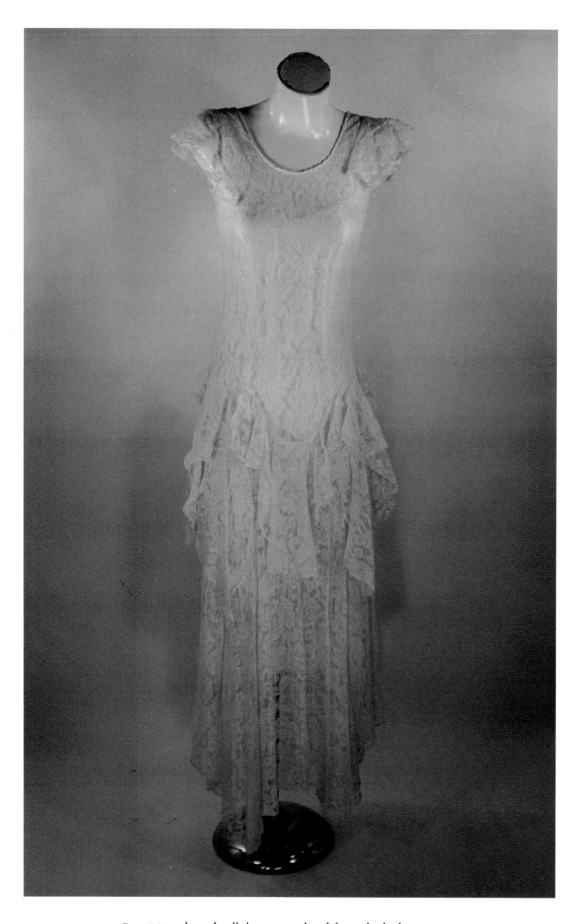

Ca. 1928 pale pink silk lace gown; lined from the bodice
down with pale pink silk; uneven hemline. *Courtesy of Lois
Fischer.*

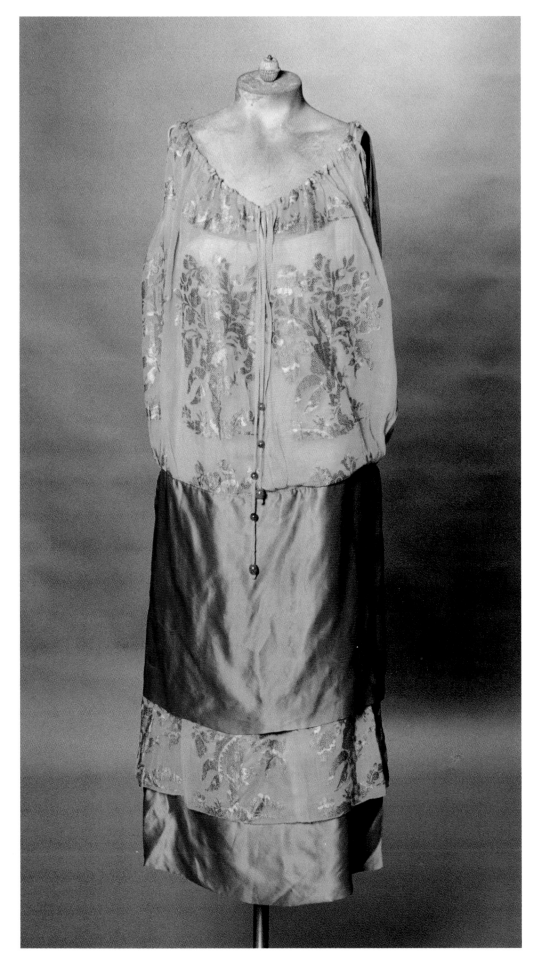

Ca. 1925 cotton sateen dress in shades of gold and lilac; gold fabric printed with mauve and metallic "tree" motif; drawstring at neckline decorated with green glass beads; labeled Callot Soeurs; Cassat provenance. *Courtesy of Mark Walsh. Photograph by Kelly Wright.*

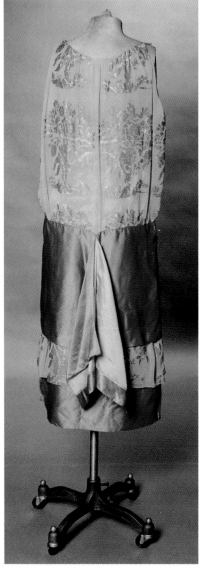

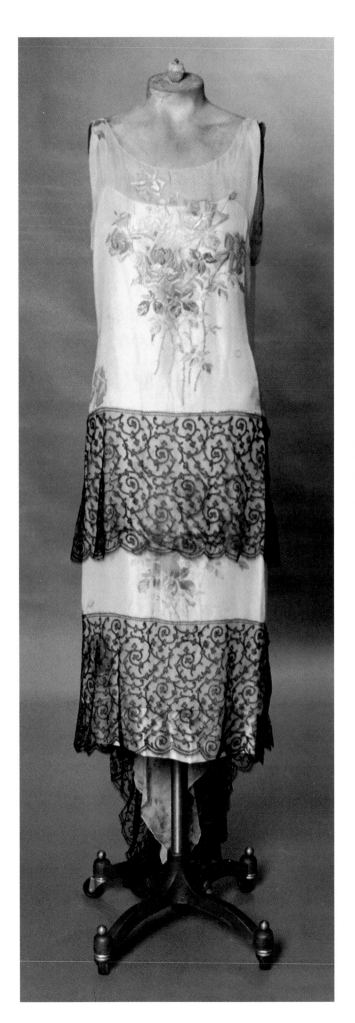

Ca. 1930 ivory silk gown printed with pink roses, pale green leaves and stems and elaborately trimmed with black Alençon lace. *Courtesy of Mark Walsh.*

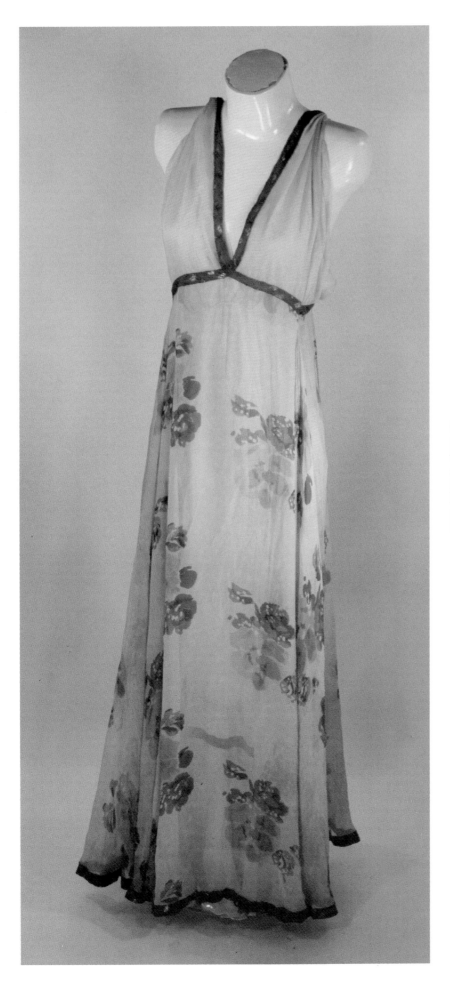

Ca. 1925 silk chiffon evening gown; lilac silk chiffon bodice, trimmed with brown and metallic silk, which is also on the slip; skirt is printed with a lilac, green, and blue floral pattern on an ivory ground; attributed to Callot Soeurs.

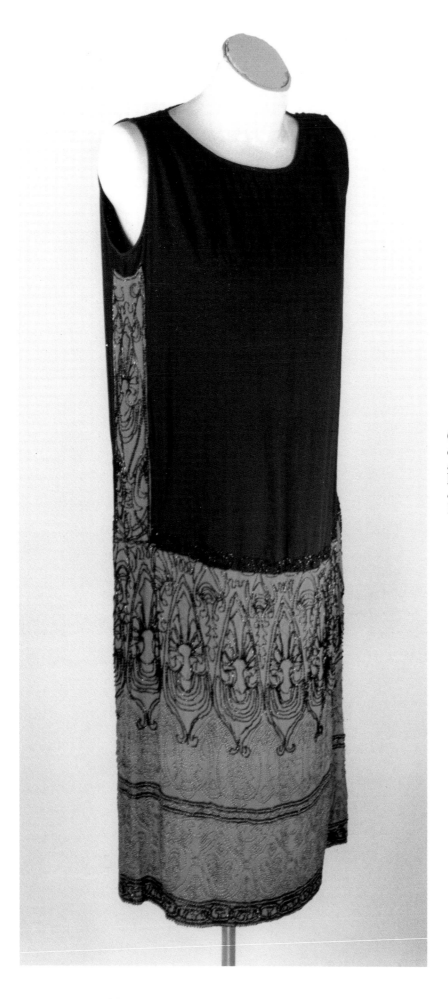

Ca. 1925 orange and black silk dress, decorated with round, gold and black glass beads; long-waisted bodice is plain; skirt is beaded all over, and up one side to armhole. Found with a matching cloche.

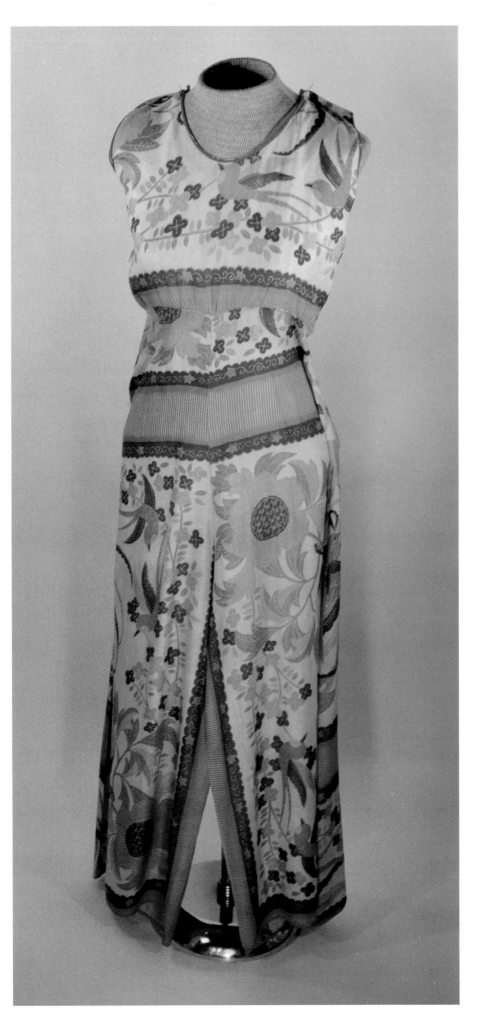

Ca. 1925 printed silk lounging pajamas, in shades of blue and tangerine on a beige background; design motif of birds and flowers.

25

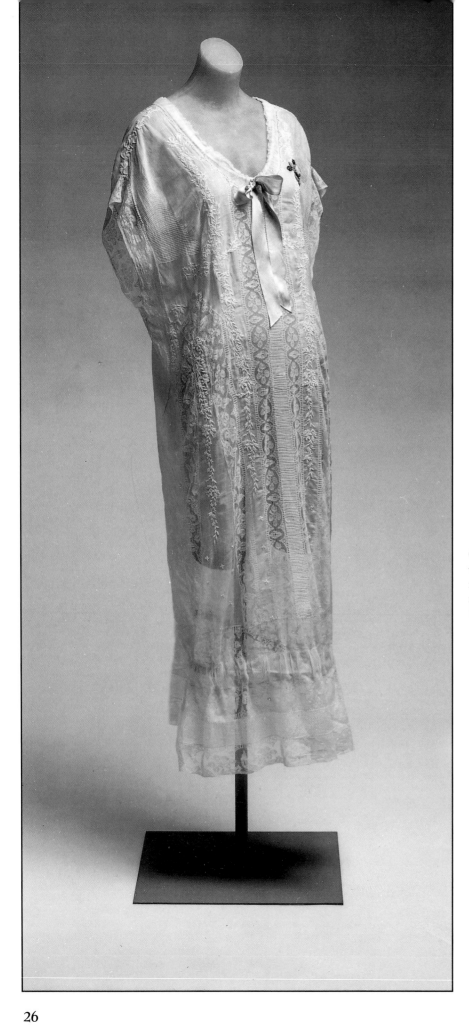

Ca. 1920 "lingerie" robe de style;
white embroidered cotton lawn with
mechlin lace, cotton net, and silk
ribbon rosettes; labeleld Boué
Soeurs. *Courtesy of Mark Walsh.*

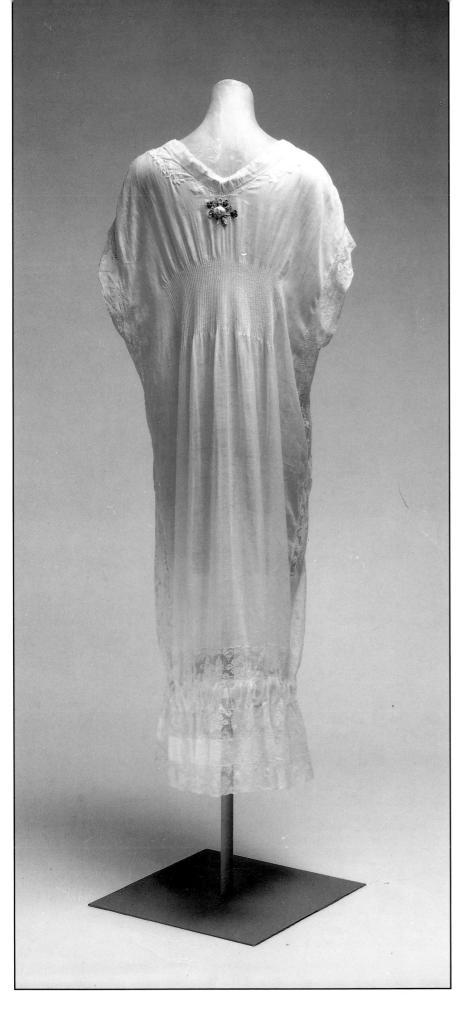

Back view of ca. 1920 "lingerie" robe de style.

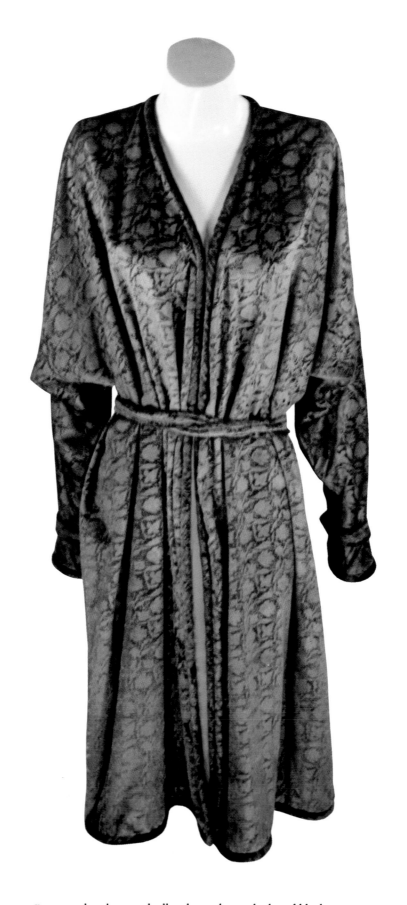

Ca. 1920 hand painted silk velvet robe in shades of black on a green background; lined with burgundy silk; labeled Mariano Fortuny, Venise. *Courtesy of the Drexel Historic Costume Collection.*

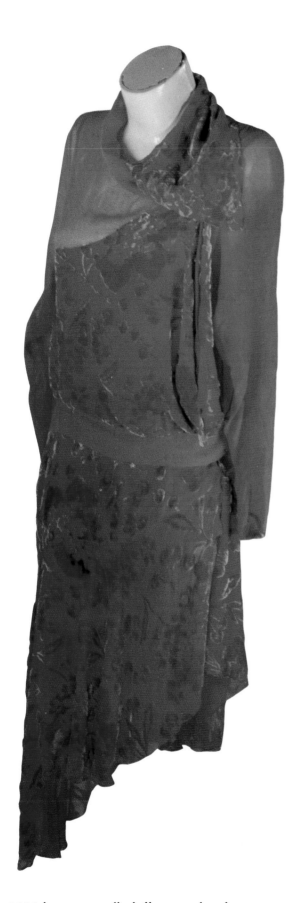

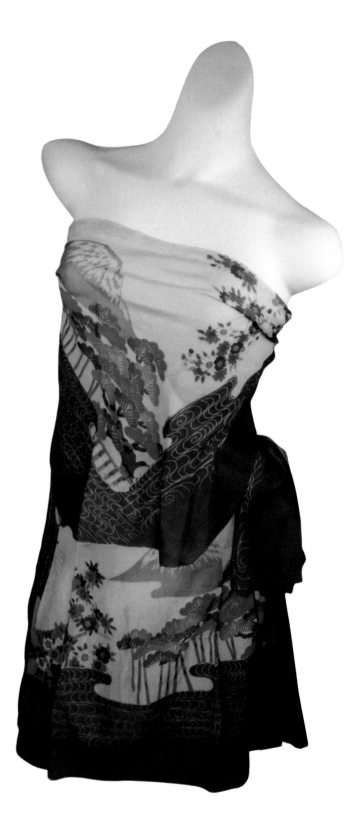

Ca. 1925 deep orange silk chiffon cut-velvet dress, uneven hemline; draped bodice; design motif of cherries, branches, and leaves.

Ca. 1925 silk shorts and "top," to be used as a scarf or halter, as shown; Oriental silk print in shades of blue, green, and deep orange on an ivory ground.

1930s

The early 1930s brought a revival of the Empress Eugénie hat and a definite trend toward tailored suits and felt hats for year round wear. Hat trimmings are simple: crown bands, aigrette feathers, or uncomplicated bows. Day dresses in rayon crepe and geometric and floral prints become popular. For late afternoon and evening wear, printed silk chiffon with petal sleeves becomes fashionable. Silk and rayon bias-cut slips and nightgowns appear, in shades of ivory, peach, pink, and ice-blue. Although many people associate the use of the zipper, or slide fastener, with the 1940s, it was actually used on men's trousers in the 1930s and by designer Elsa Schiaparelli in Paris in 1933 for high fashion apparel (*Fairchild's Dictionary of Fashion, 2nd Edition*). However, the zipper was not widely used in skirts, gowns, and dresses until the early 1940s.

Ca. 1930 printed silk chiffon afternoon dress, with a geometric "feather" pattern in shades of white, green, blue, and rose on a black background; same material belt.

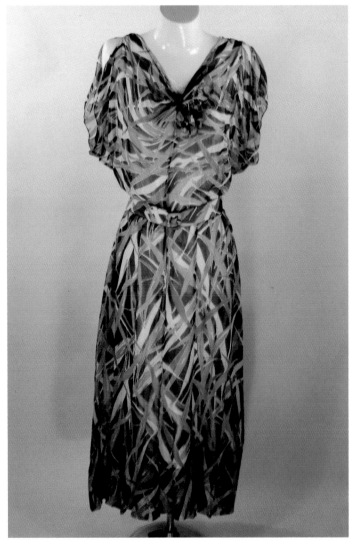

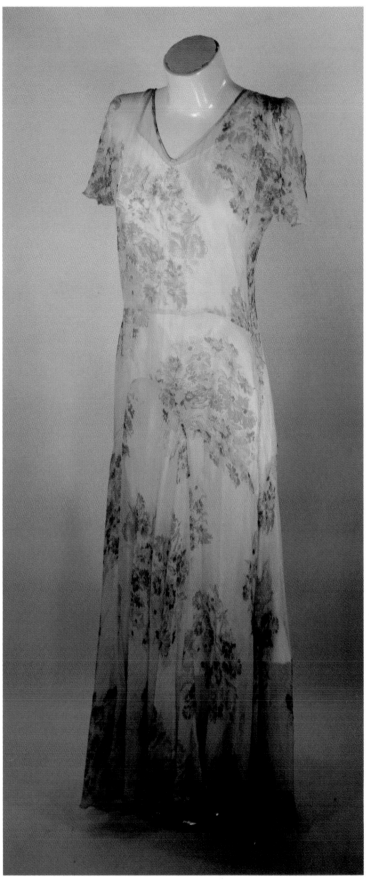

Ca. 1930 floral printed silk chiffon dress, in shades of blue and orange on a beige background; cut on the bias; cape sleeves.

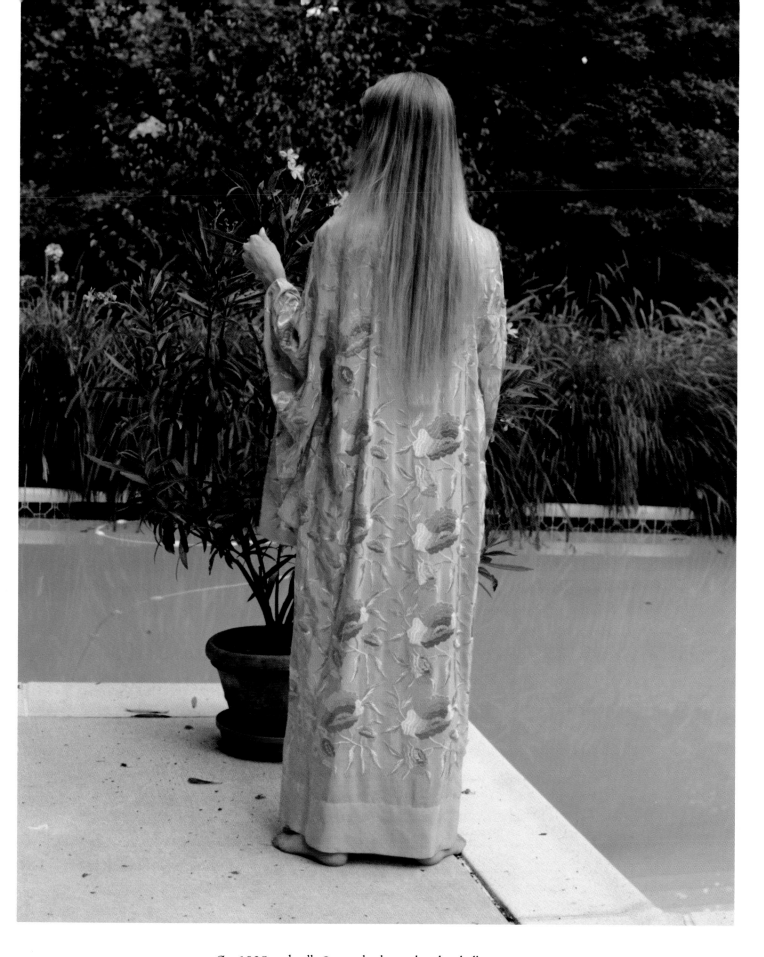

Ca. 1935 pink silk Oriental robe, embroidered all over in a
floral design in shades of rose and moss green. *Modeled by
Marcie Behanna.*

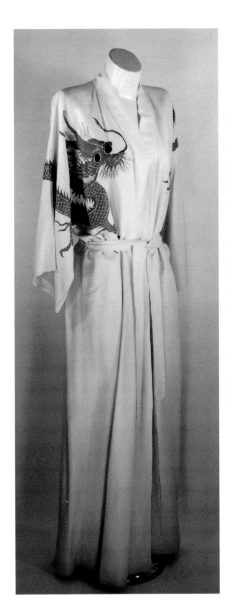

Ca. 1930 raw silk Oriental robe, embroidered in blue silk thread with a dragon, which goes entirely around the robe. An exceptional piece!

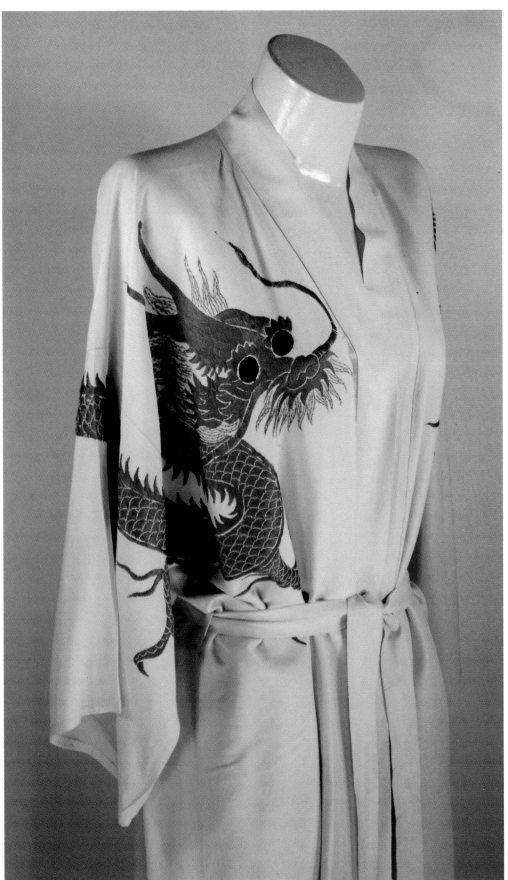

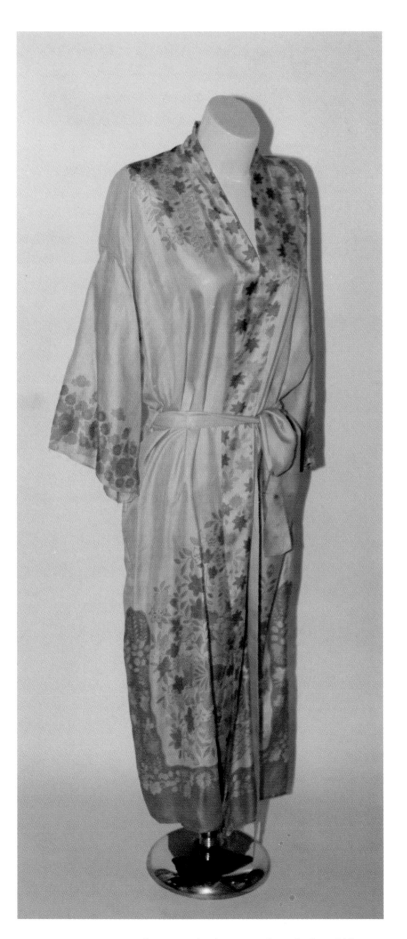

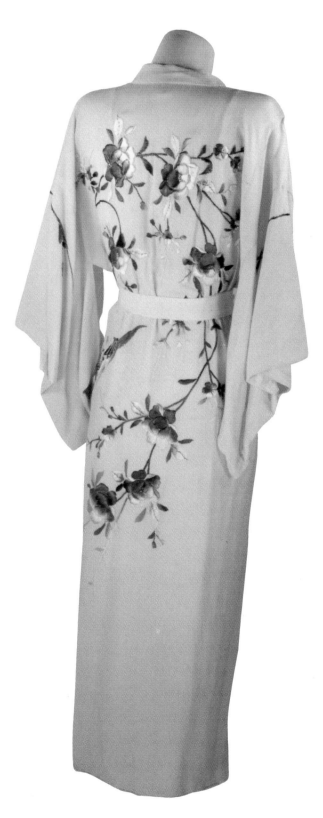

Ca. 1935 ivory silk Oriental robe, printed in shades of blue, green, and orange; ivory silk sash.

Ca. 1935 ivory crepe Oriental robe, embroidered in blue and white threads in a floral motif.

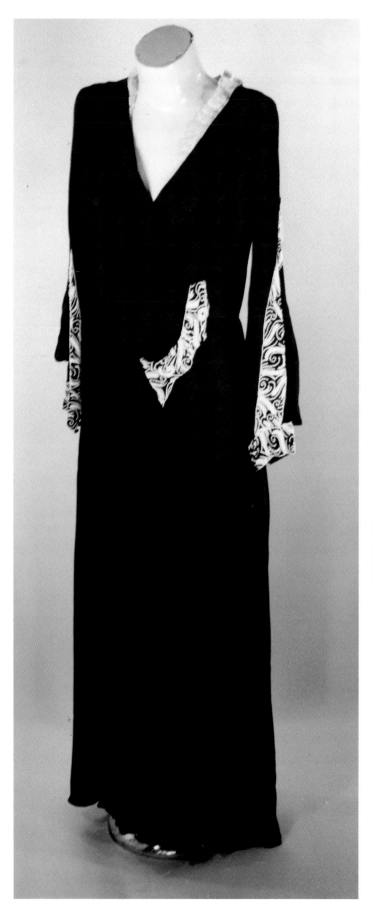

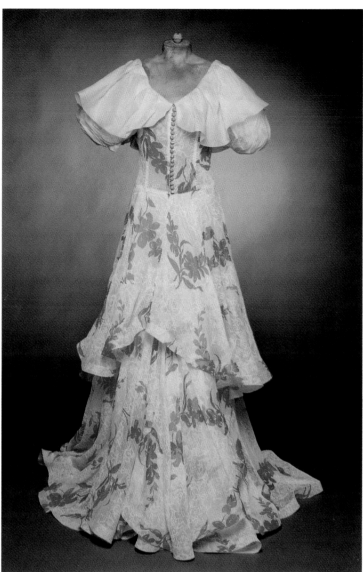

Ca. 1930 "Garden Party Dress" of two-tiered cotton organdy printed with a red and white floral motif; fabric covered buttons from the neckline to the waist, cape collar which extends over large, puffed sleeves; labeled Maggy Rouff. A fascinating dress! *Courtesy of Mark Walsh. Photograph by Kelly Wright*

Ca. 1930 black silk crepe gown, decorated with round, white glass beads.

Ca. 1938 black silk, tissue taffeta evening gown; with lilac silk velvet waist trim and shoulder straps, studded with rhinestones; labeled Copy of Original Suzanne Talbot, 14 rue royale, paris. *Courtesy of Karen Augusta.*

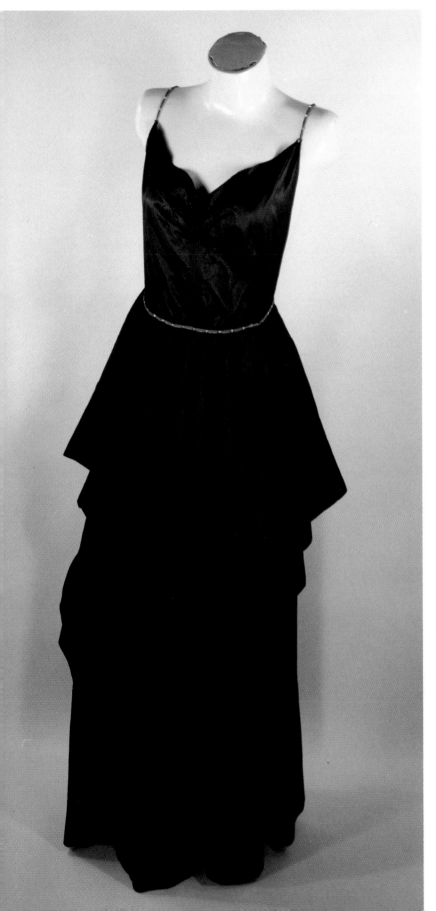

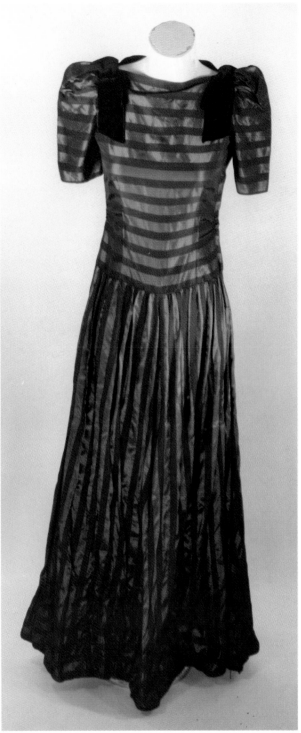

Ca. 1935 burgundy and black iridescent taffeta gown, with a black silk velvet bow on each shoulder; labeled Margie Joy Juniors. *A gift from Margaret Heath Smith.*

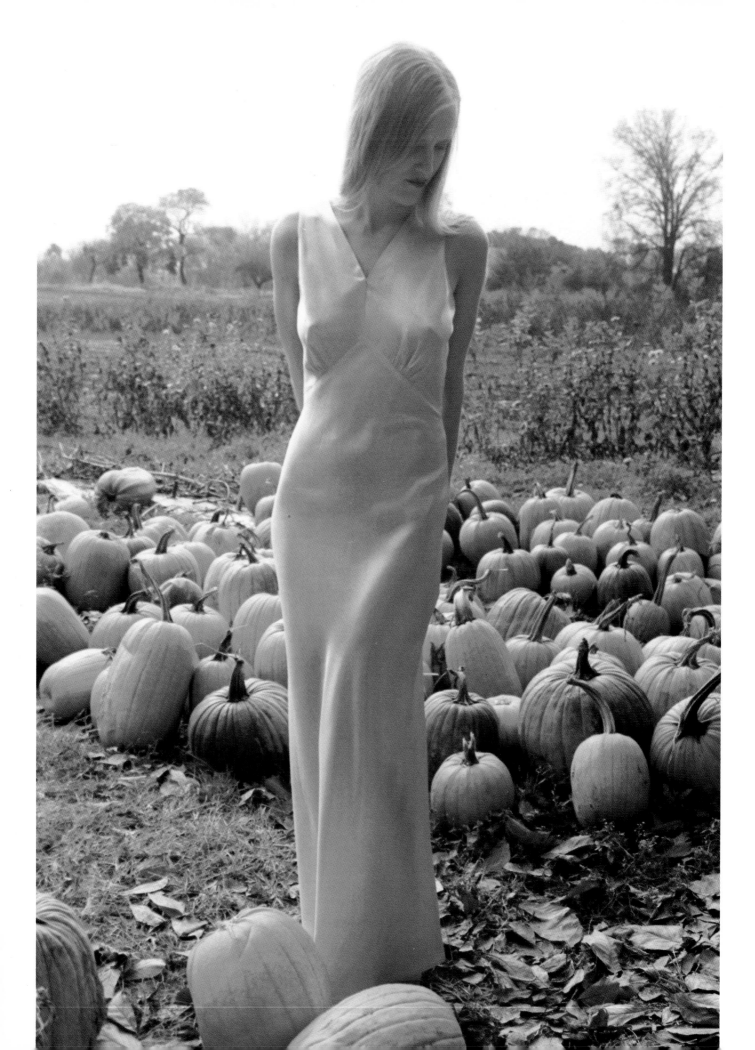

Ca. 1935 rose rayon satin night-gown; bias cut with wide shoulder straps. *Modeled by Marcie Behanna.*

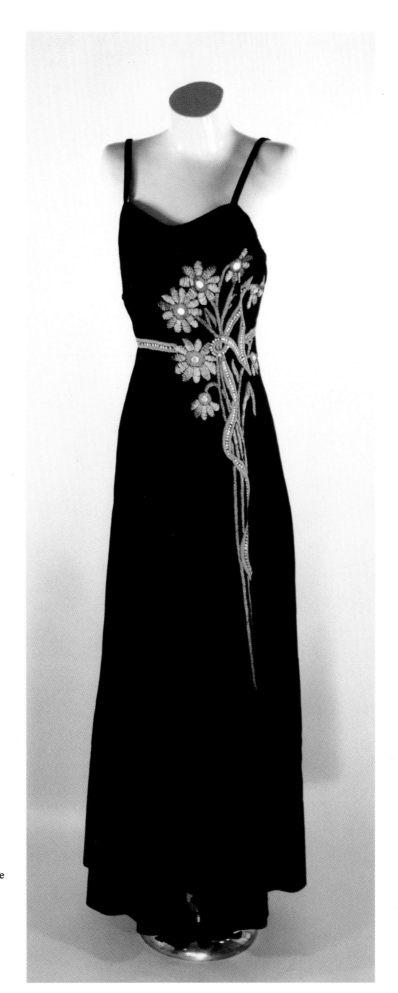

Ca. 1930 black silk velvet gown, elaborately embroidered in a floral motif in shades of tangerine and tan; floral centers are sequins; waistline is dotted with rhinestones, as is much of the embroidered "ribbon" around the flowers. Truly a work of art!

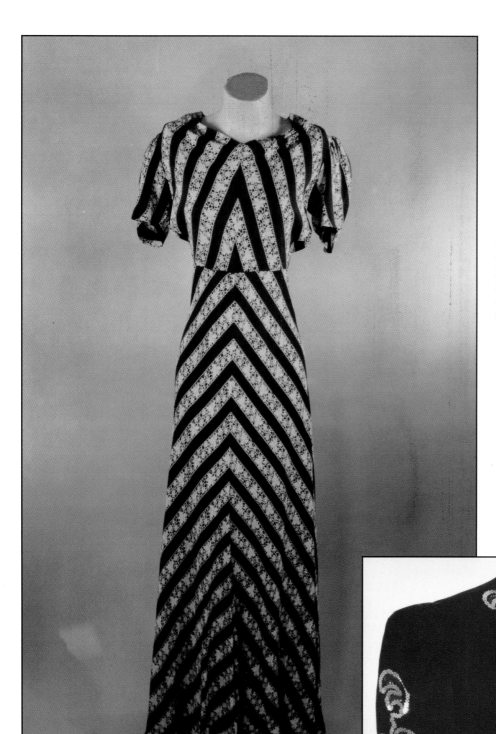

Ca. 1935 black silk gown, printed with ivory "lace;" entirely open back, with small, same-material covered buttons at waist. The concept of "printed lace" is most unusual.

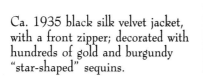

Ca. 1935 black silk velvet jacket, with a front zipper; decorated with hundreds of gold and burgundy "star-shaped" sequins.

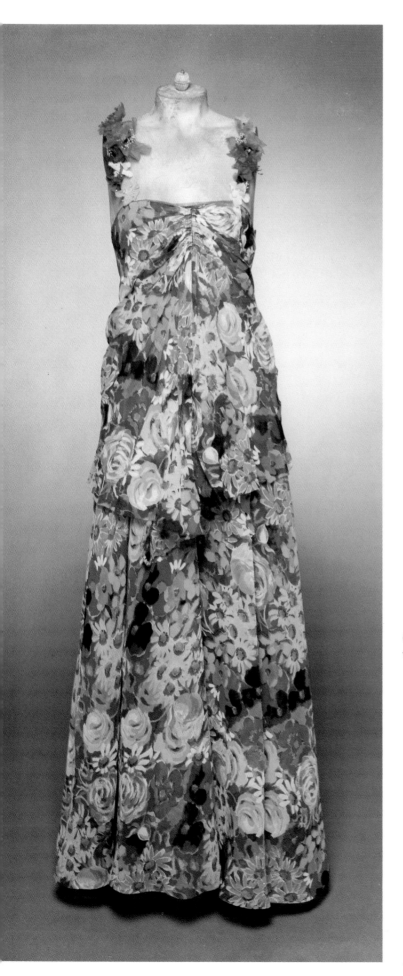

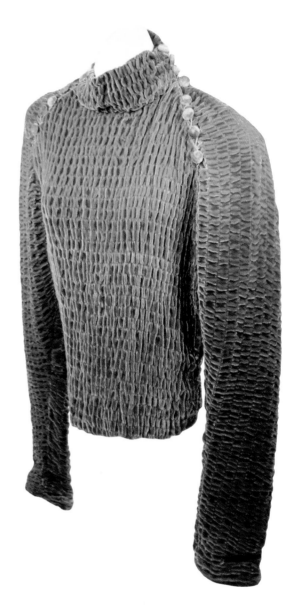

Ca. 1930 green silk velvet top, smocked all over; buttoned with five covered buttons across each shoulder.

Ca. 1930 silk gown printed all over in a floral motif in shades of blue, yellow, red, green, pink, and gold; silk flowers in shades of blue, yellow, red, and white decorate the straps; labeled Maggy Rouff. A structurally fascinating gown with fabric as dense and beautiful as a flower garden! *Courtesy of Mark Walsh. Photograph by Kelly Wright.*

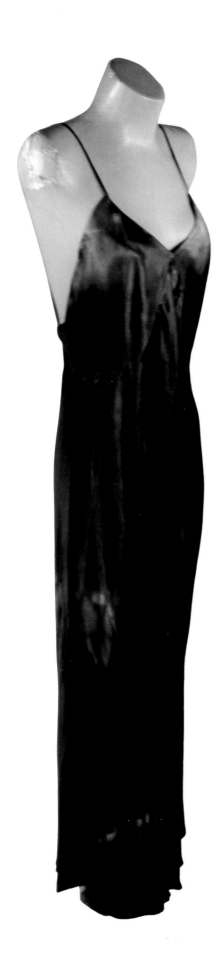

Ca. 1930 purple silk "tie-dyed" slip, cut on the bias; straps show evidence that the fabric was "tie-dyed" before the garment was made; labeled Barbizon, Paris.

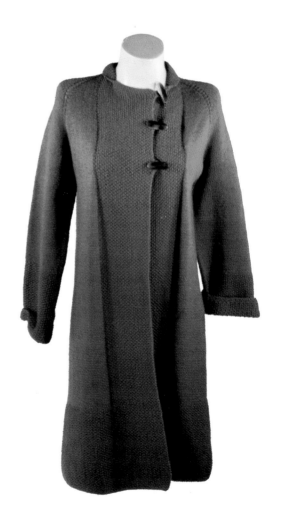

Ca. 1930 brown knitted sweater/coat, appropriate for golfing; with three, large Bakelite buttons.

Ca. 1930 rayon print dress in shades of burgundy, blue and yellow; grosgrain ribbon trim.

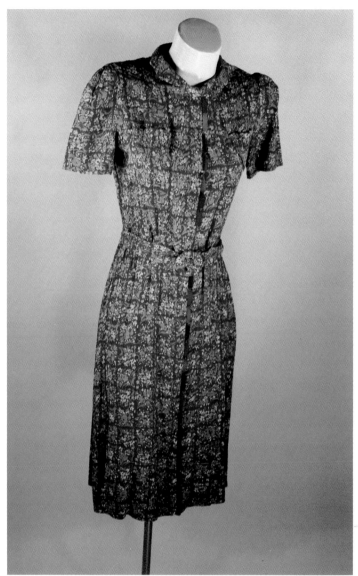

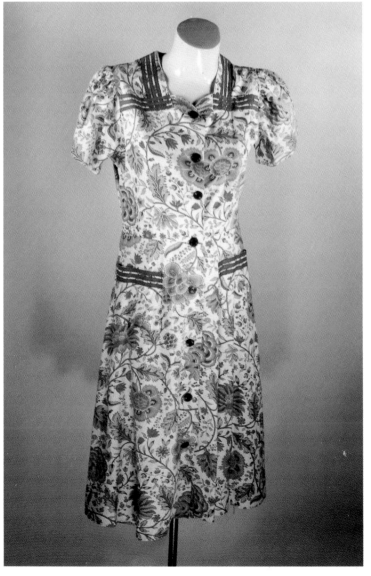

Ca. 1935 cotton day dress, in a colorful print of lilac, green, and burgundy on a white background; labeled Riviera Modes. Acquired in Jersey Shore, Pennsylvania, with approximately two-hundred additional dresses of its type, from the estate of a needle-trades worker.

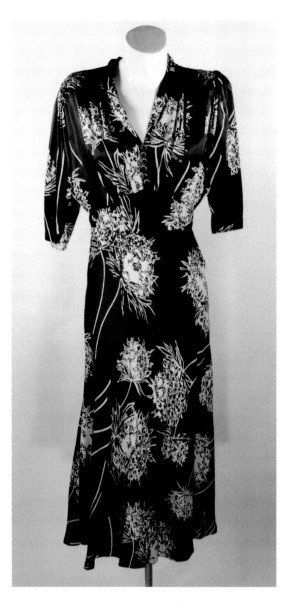

Ca. 1930 navy blue silk with hand painted floral pattern in ivory; black glass buttons, encircled with rhinestones. Acquired in Paris; unknown couturier.

Ca. 1935 dress of rust, textured crepe that is heat-set in a crimped manner; two-tiered with front buttons which open only to the waist; labeled College Princess, Original Model.

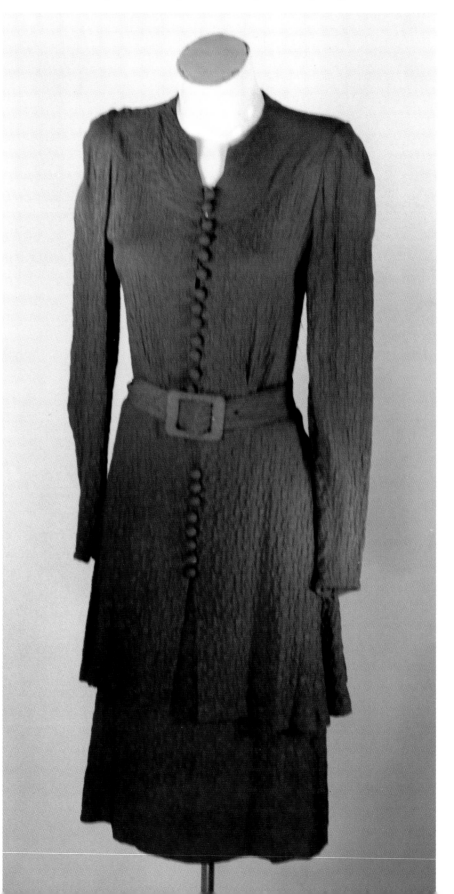

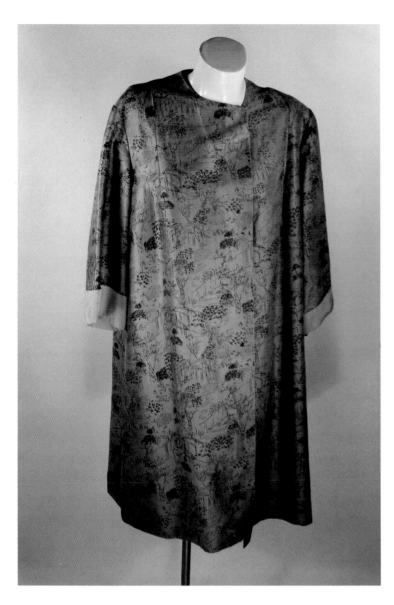

Ca. 1930 Oriental silk brocade wrap coat in mauve and black; lined with tan silk.

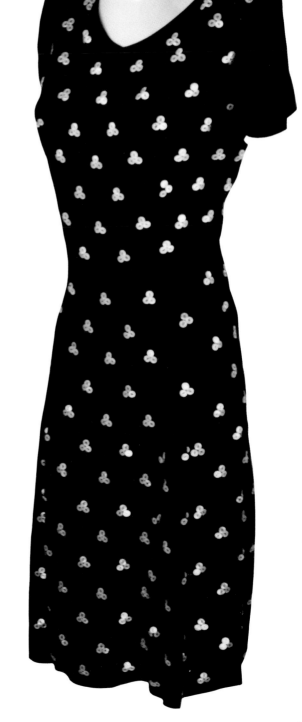

Ca. 1930 black silk crepe dress, front decorated all over with clusters of white, mother-of-pearl buttons; each cluster has three buttons.

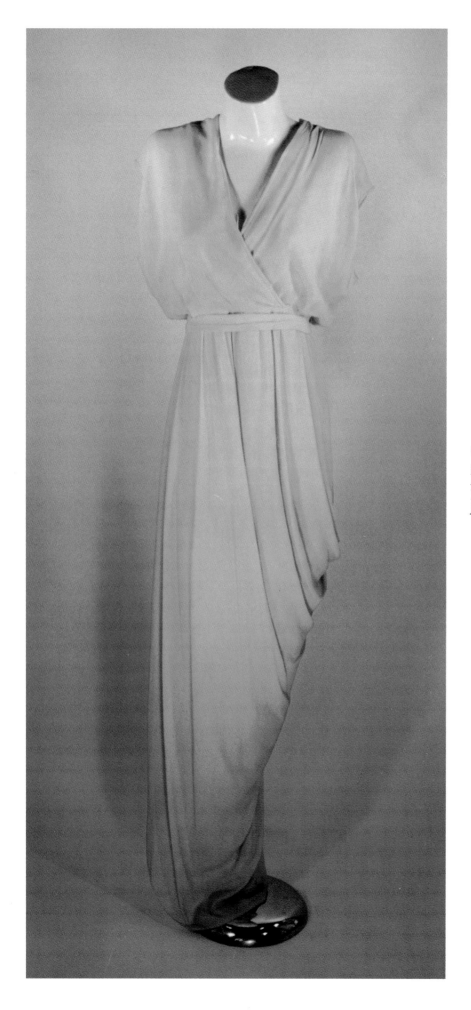

Ca. 1930 softly draped yellow silk
gown; lined in sheer, ivory silk;
labeled Modele Molyneux, 14, Rue
Royale. *Courtesy of the Drexel
Historic Costume Collection.*

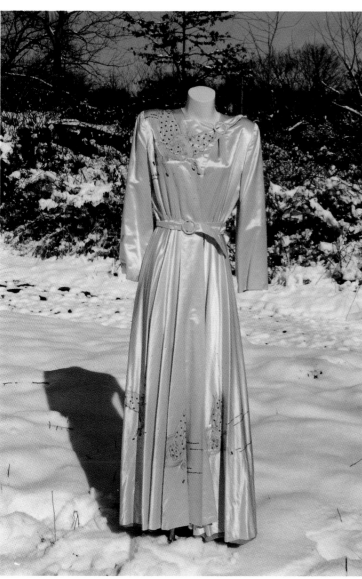

The suits, jackets, and coats of the 1940s are perhaps the most beautifully tailored in fashion history. I personally consider the 1940s jackets to be, in the fashion world, comparable in quality to Philadelphia Chippendale furniture! Covered buttons, patch pockets, with flaps, lapels of all descriptions, garments in crepe and gabardine decorated with sequins, soutache, and beading are all characteristic of the 1940s. The restrictions of Act L85, the U.S. government wartime order limiting the hem measurement of a skirt to 72" around and the trimming material in each dress to half a yard, was less of a burden to some designers than to others. Rayon prints have an asymmetrical look, and the bias-cut, a line cut diagonally across the grain of the fabric, becomes the design of choice for evening gowns. Millinery is as structurally diverse as it ever gets, with felt trimming coming into vogue, possibly due to the wartime restrictions on trimmings.

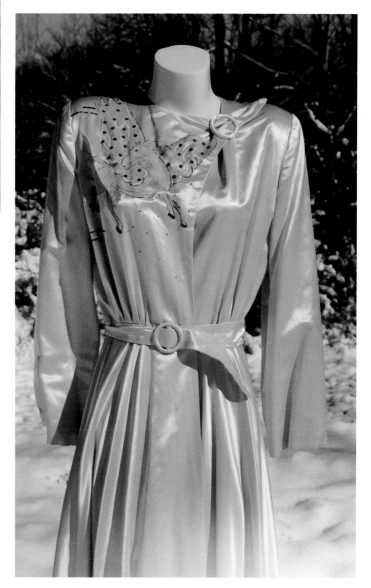

Ca. 1940 ivory silk satin robe, hand painted with a "Pegasus" motif, in shades of blue and rose; additionally decorated with red, glass bugle beads, and red sequins; lined with rose silk chiffon; signed on silk garment bag, custom made for the robe, Cloud Swept by Madelyn Whiting. This is a most unusual piece, because it was given a "title" by its creator.

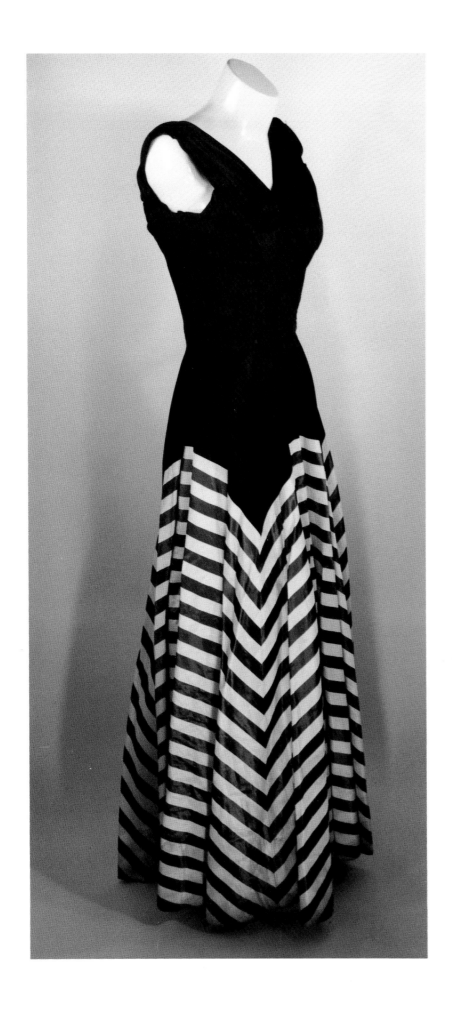

Ca. 1940 taffeta gown; black bodice and skirt to hipline; then balance of skirt is of ivory and black taffeta; some gathering on bodice. When flat on the floor, the top of the gown is a perfect square in the center of yards of material. Structurally incredible!

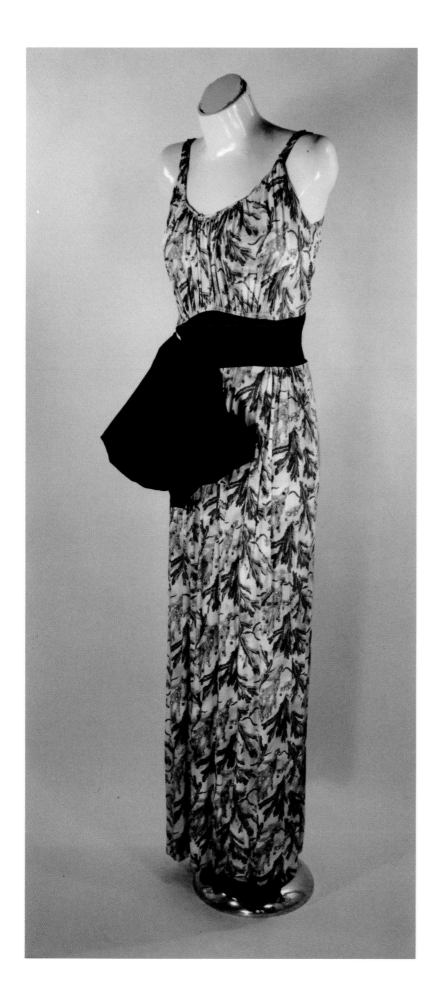

Ca. 1940 silk crepe evening gown, printed in a leaf motif, in shades of green and mauve; studded all over with green glass set in brass; silk taffeta midriff and large bow at waist; labeled Esther Pomerantz (a Philadelphia retailer).

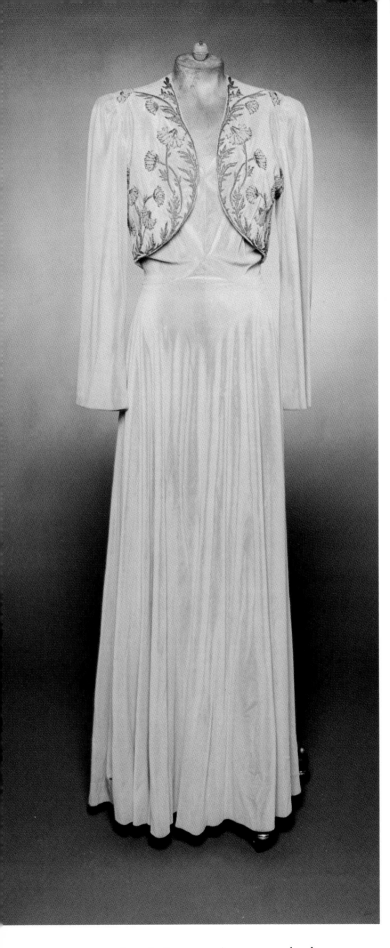

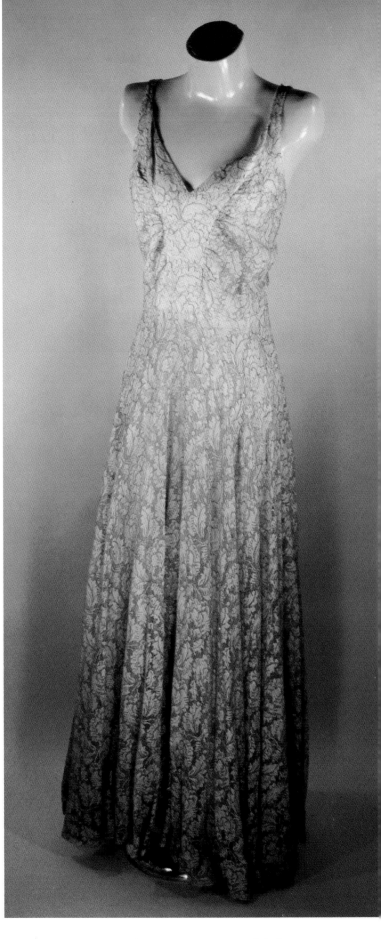

Ca. 1940 pink washed cotton velvet gown and jacket, embroidered with gold poppies; labeled Schiaparelli. *Courtesy of Mark Walsh. Photograph by Kelly Wright.*

Ca. 1945 ivory cotton lace evening gown; "solid" lace areas are edged with black thread; lined with ivory taffeta; labeled Eisenberg & Sons Original. *Courtesy of Karen Augusta.*

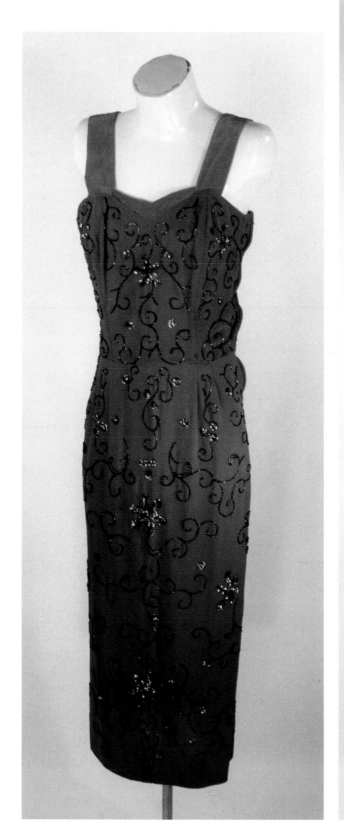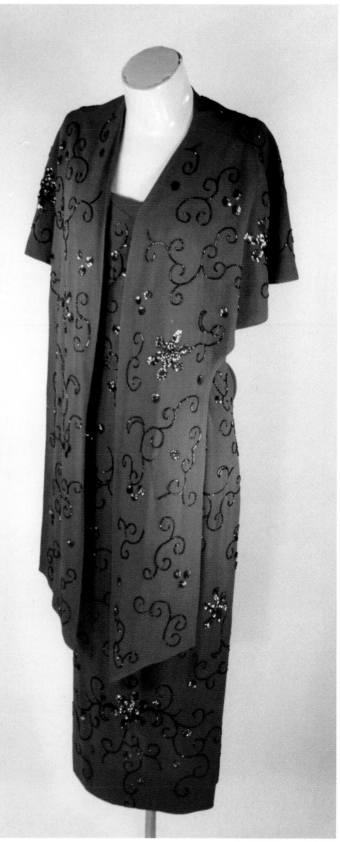

Ca. 1940 gray crepe gown, decorated with gray iridescent
sequins; red silk velvet straps and bodice detailing; matching
stole. This gown belonged to Gracie Boyajian Young, who
was the first Miss Atlantic City, New Jersey (Queen's Court,
1921).

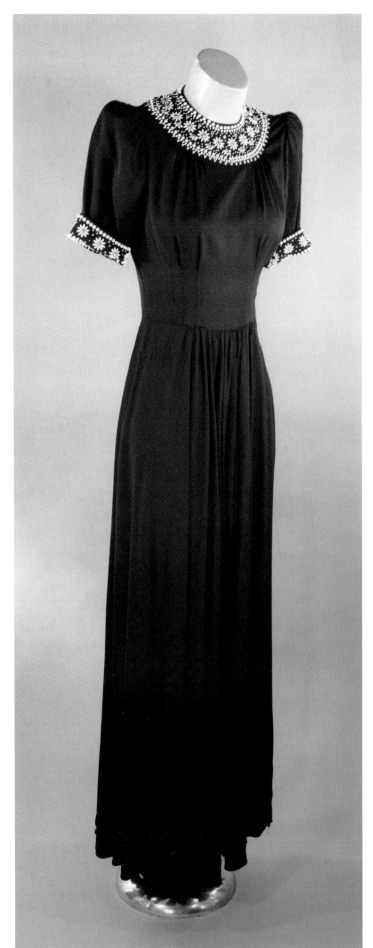

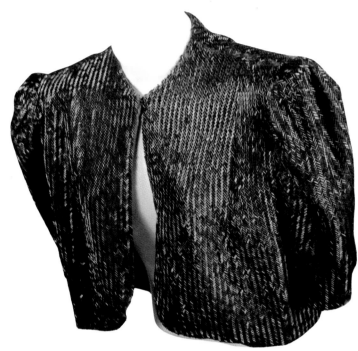

Ca. 1940 burgundy beaded dinner jacket; beaded all over in the "herringbone pattern;" lined with burgundy silk.

Ca. 1940 black crepe gown; collar and cuffs elaborately decorated with white, glass beads, in a floral motif.

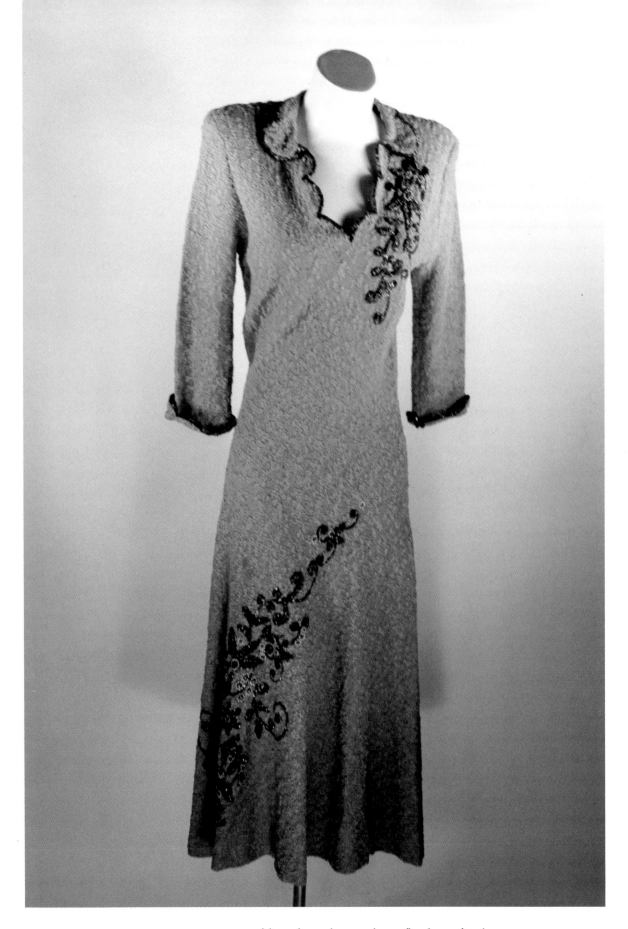

Ca. 1940 tan wool knit dress, decorated in a floral motif with copper bugle beads at the back, the front, and at the collar and cuffs; labeled Hand Knit Elegance by Diane, Beverly Hills, Calif., 100% wool-imported yarns.

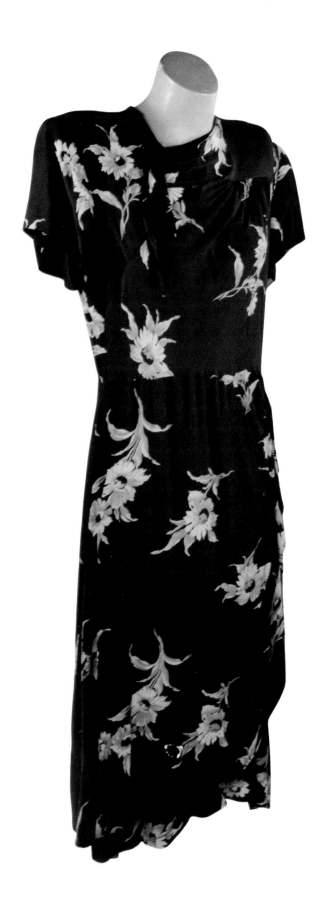

Ca. 1940 rayon print dress, in brown with a yellow floral design; elaborate draping and gathering of bodice and skirt.

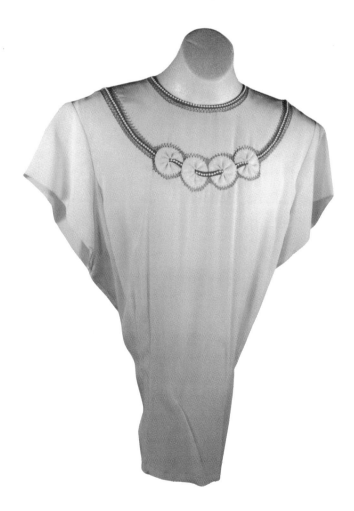

Ca. 1940 beige silk crepe blouse, decorated with orange stitching and round, white glass beads.

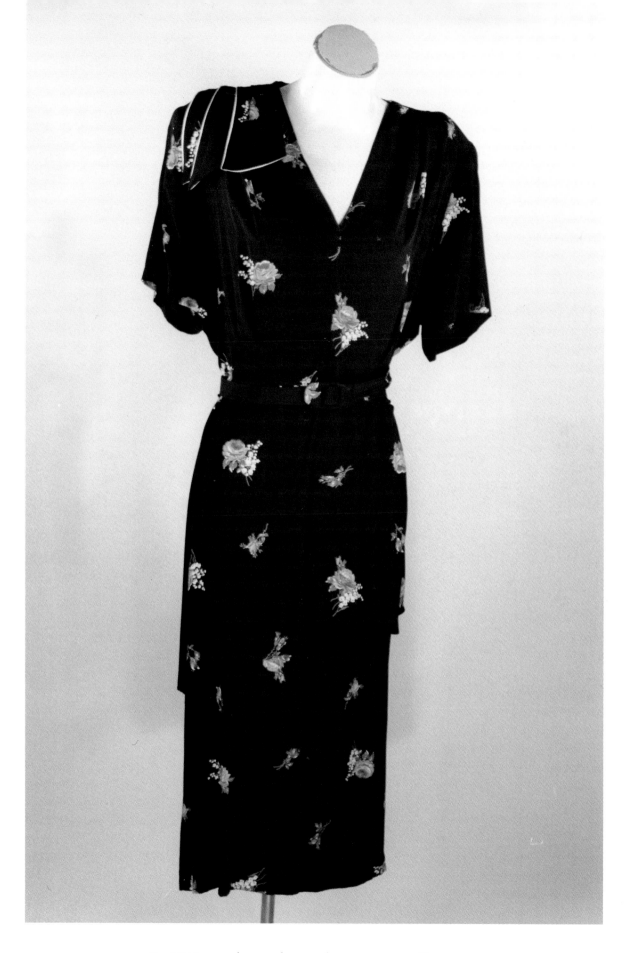

Ca. 1940 printed rayon dress, with roses on a navy blue
background; three overlapping shoulder "flaps" and a draped
hipline.

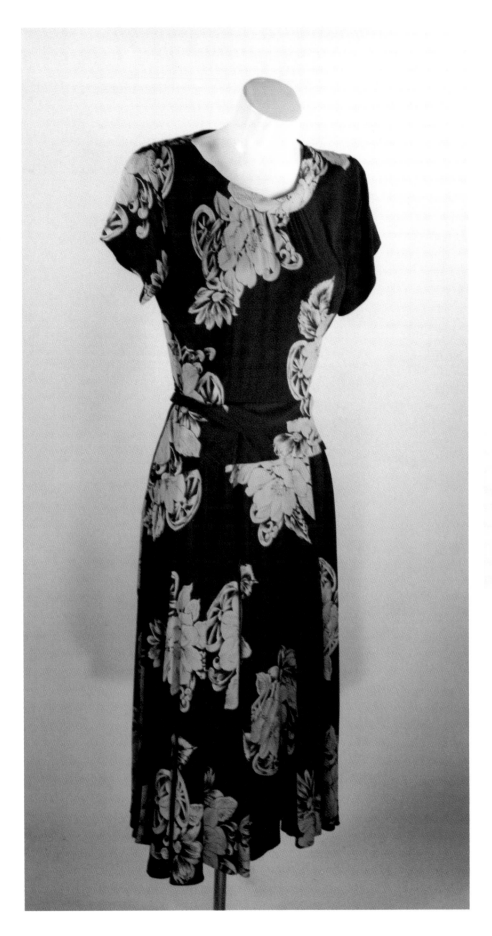

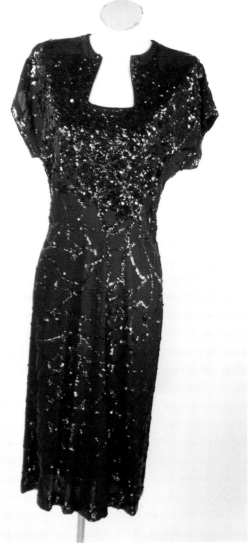

Ca. 1940 black crepe dress, decorated front and back with black sequins; keyhole neckline; labeled An Aldrich Original.

Ca. 1940 black silk crepe dress, decorated with mauve sequins in geometric patterns, on collar, bodice, and all over sleeves; labeled Eisenberg Originals.

Ca. 1940 printed rayon dress, in shades of pale aqua and mauve on a navy blue background; draped bodice.

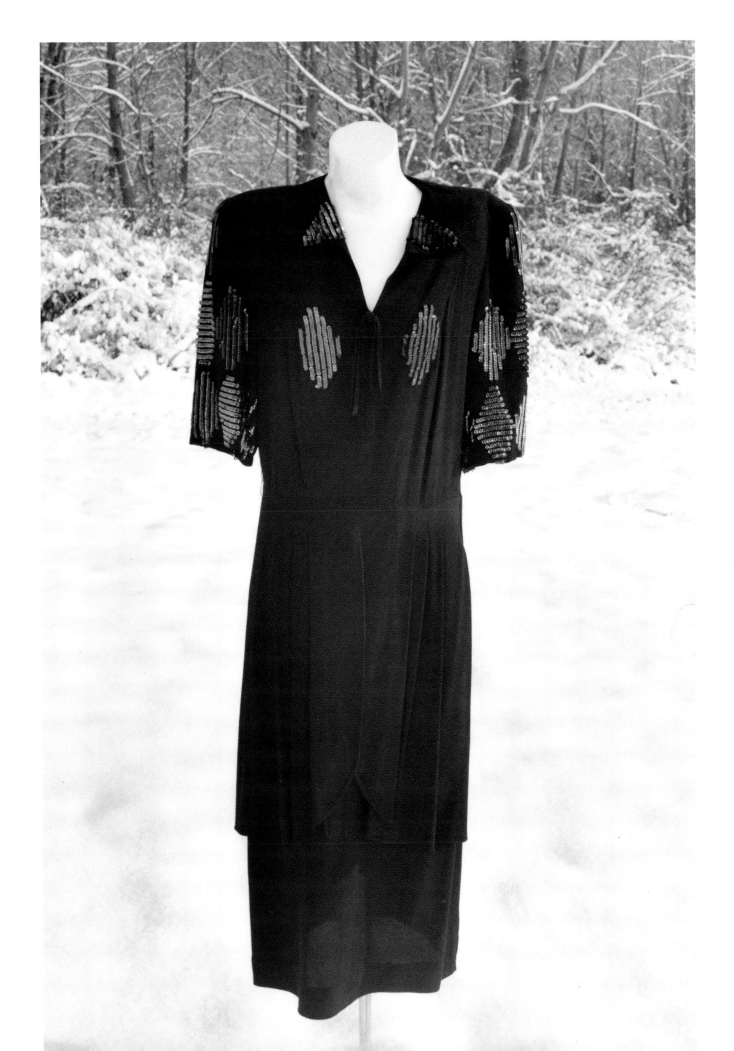

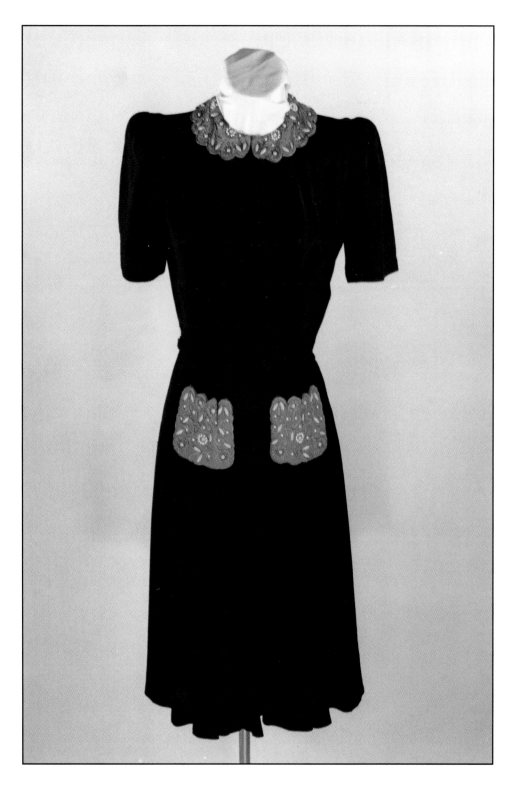

Ca. 1940 black crepe dress, with tangerine crepe front pockets and collar, embroidered with gold thread and decorated with turquoise glass beads and small synthetic pearls. This dress is fascinating in terms of the contrasting colors and decorative detail. *Courtesy of Lois Fischer.*

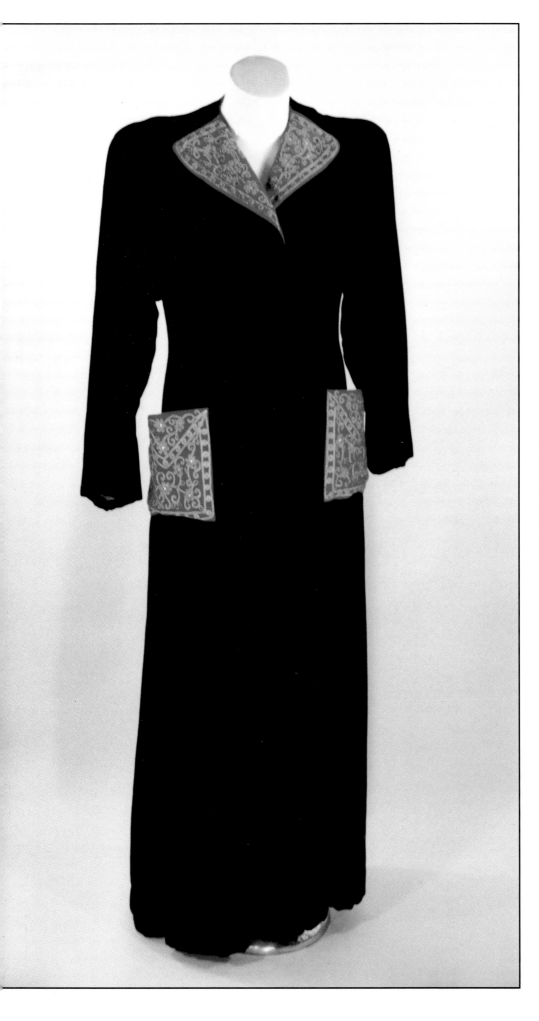

Ca. 1940 black silk velvet evening coat, with red flannel pockets and lapels, embroidered with gold thread and studded with rhinestones; lined with red silk taffeta; labeled Hess Brothers, Allentown. An exceptionally beautiful design for evening!

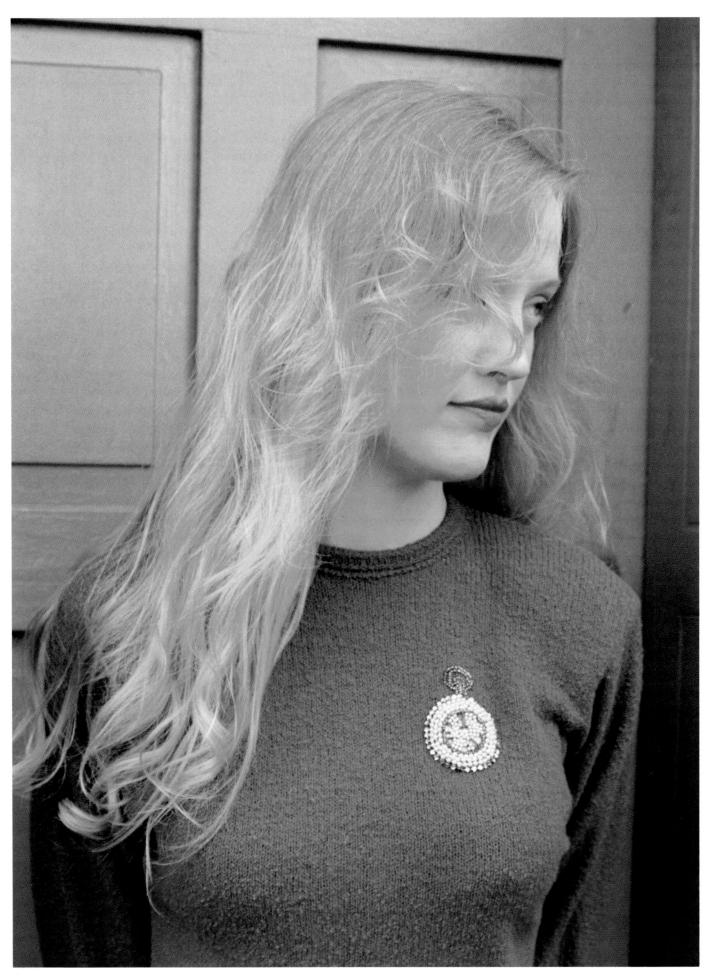

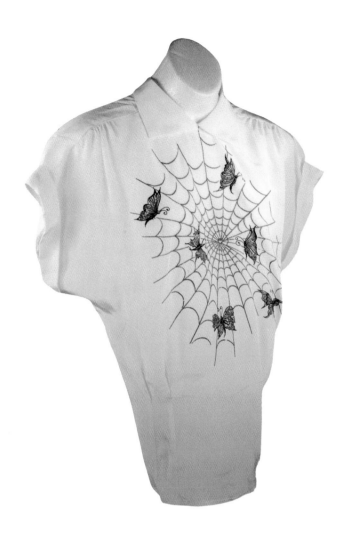

Ca. 1945 white rayon crepe blouse, printed with a "web" full of colorful butterflies.

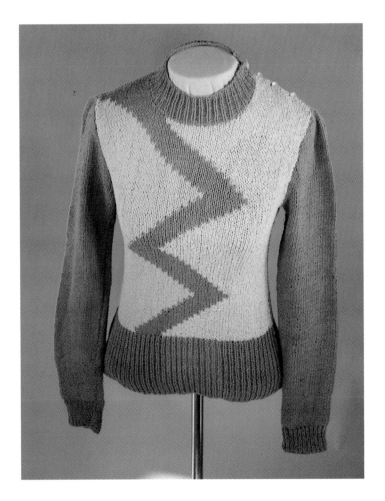

Ca. 1945 teal blue wool knit top, decorated with a "pocket watch" made of silver glass beads and seed pearls. *Modeled by Marcie Behanna.*

Ca. 1940 mauve, lilac, and ivory-metallic sweater with a zig-zag design; mother-of-pearl buttons across one shoulder; solid lilac back.

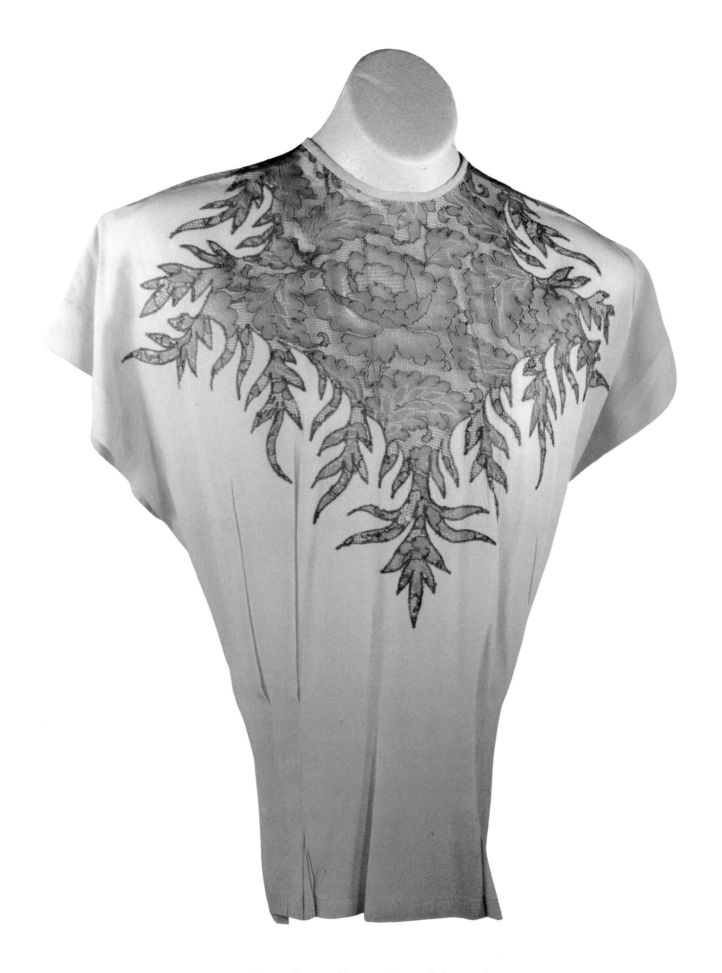

Ca. 1940 beige silk crepe blouse with tan silk lace appliqué.

1950s

Straight skirts, bubble skirts, bouffant skirts, pleated skirts, dirndl skirts, and crinolines all become popular in the 1950s. The image of fashion becomes more feminine. Shoulder pads disappear. The little black dress emerges. Variations of the picture hat appear--wide-brimmed felts and straws that look fashionable with princess-line dresses and bolero jackets. These are the days of the poodle skirt and the prom gown!

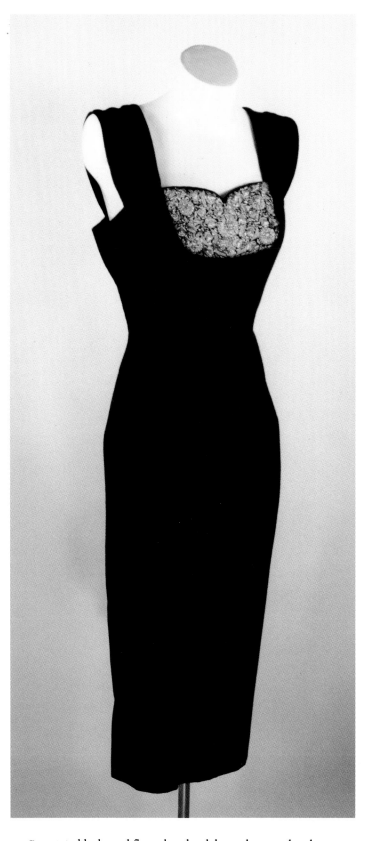

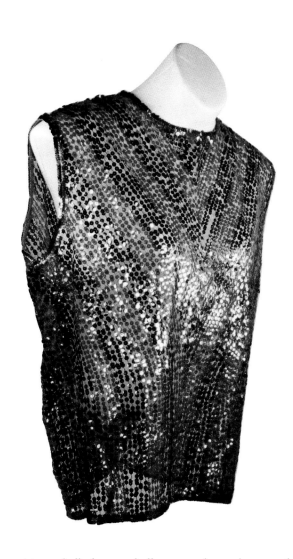

Ca. 1955 net shell, decorated all over in charcoal gray and fuchsia sequins; labeled Hand Made in France.

Ca. 1950 black wool flannel cocktail dress, decorated with elaborate gold braid in a floral motif; flowers' centers of white beads; labeled Glenn Thomas; Designed by Betty Soehngen For Glenn Thomas Co., Inc.

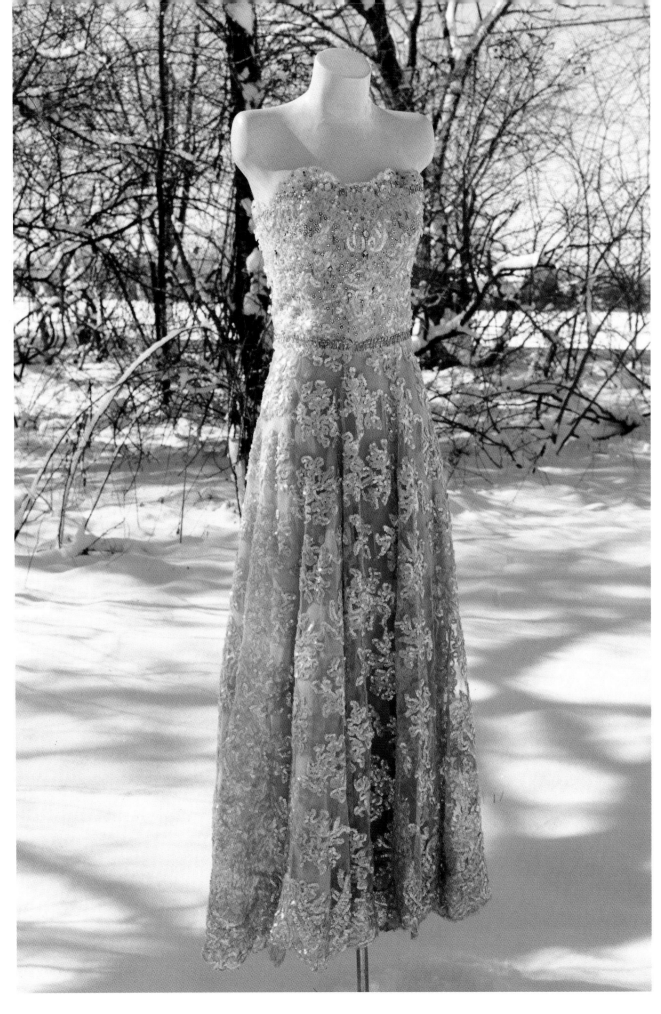

Ca. 1950 ivory net strapless gown, elaborately embroidered all over with iridescent ivory sequins; bodice additionally decorated with rhinestones; bodice lined in ivory silk; skirt has two additional layers of net. Every sequin on the gown was hand sewn; each rhinestone hand set!

Dated 1952, black tissue taffeta gown, with an entire bodice and sleeves in handmade black silk lace; "yards and yards"of black silk tissue taffeta make up two underskirts, one of which is trimmed at the bottom with black silk lace, identical to that used for the bodice; the final layer is a stiffened net petticoat, which is lined with silk; labeled Bergdorf Goodman, On The Plaza, New York.

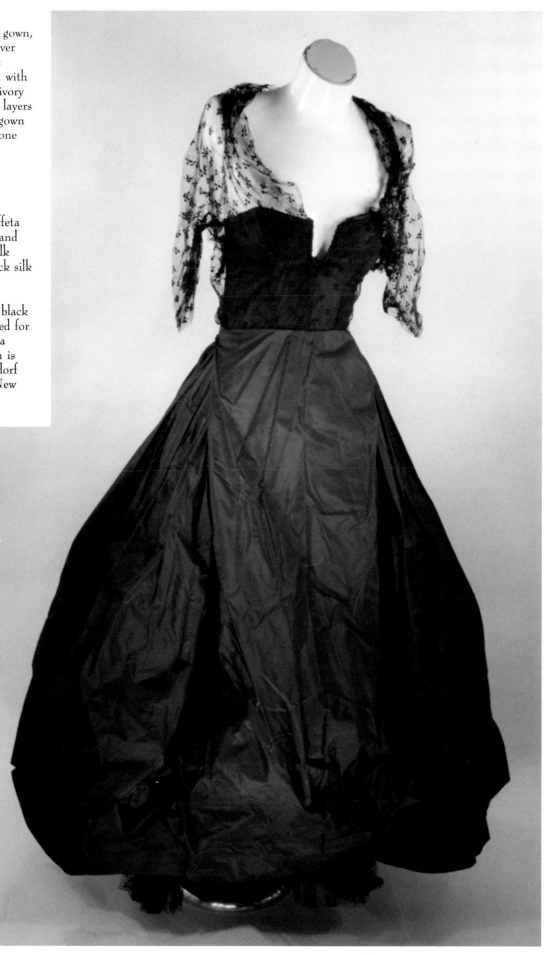

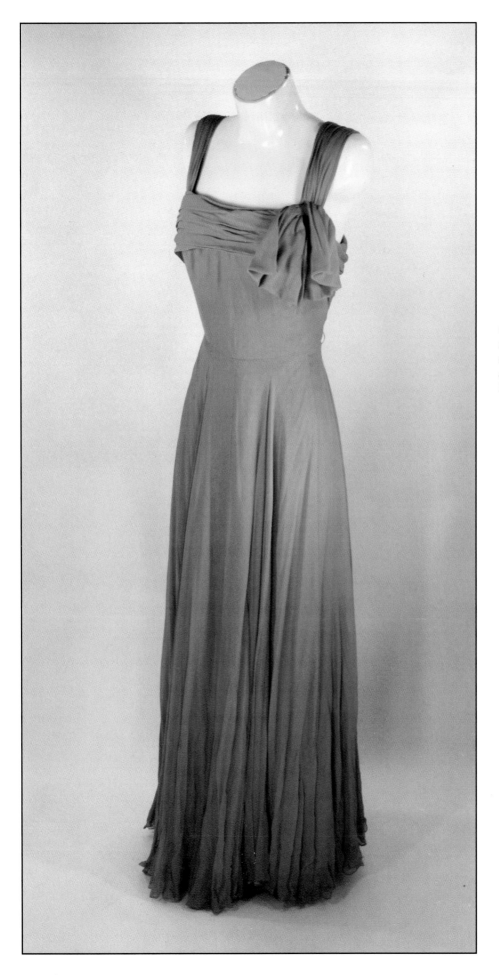

Ca. 1955 evening gown, made of many layers of gray-blue over aqua silk chiffon, with an underdress of aqua silk crepe; labeled Nan Duskin.

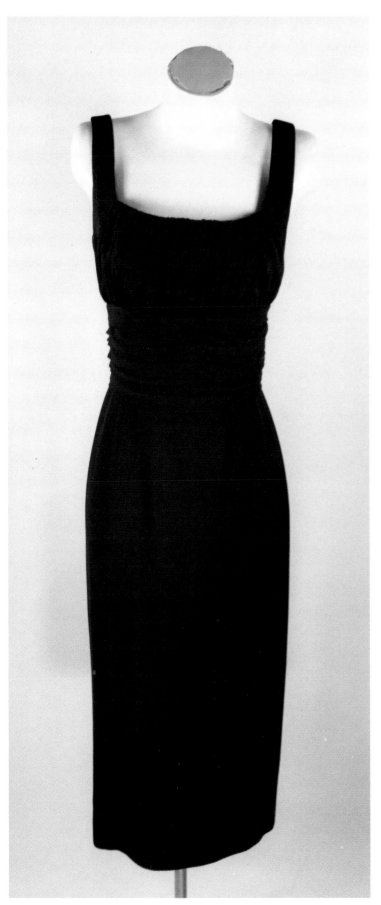

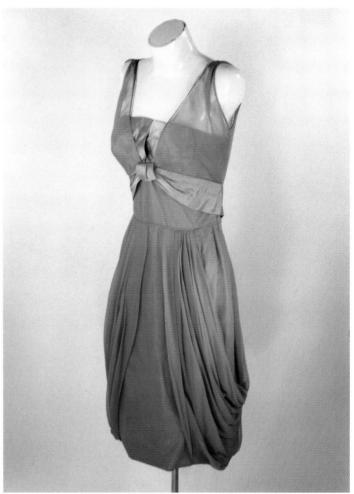

Ca. 1955 blue, silk chiffon cocktail dress; sheath skirt, draped with silk chiffon; silk satin "empire" effect on bodice; lined with taffeta; labeled Mignon, Paris, New York.

Ca. 1950 black, silk crepe cocktail dress; labeled GiGi Young, New York.

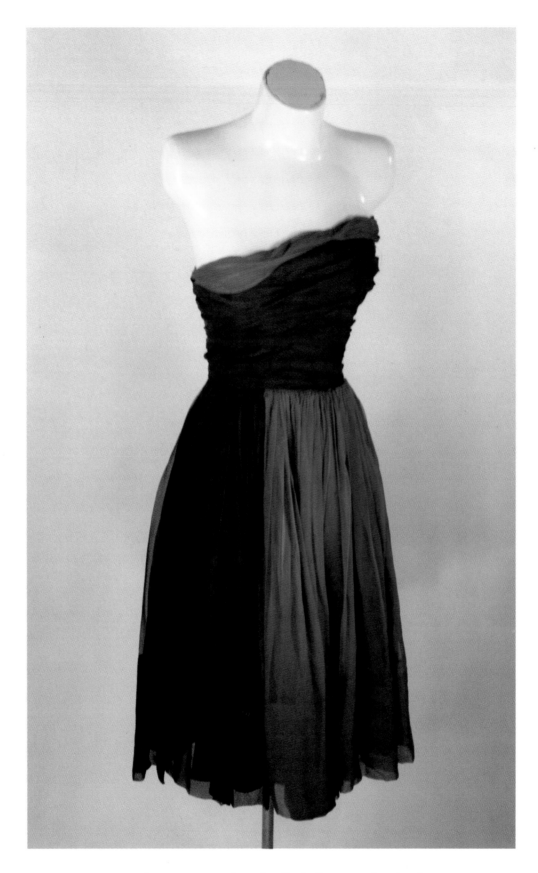

Dated 1952 green and purple silk chiffon gown; lined with mauve silk; labeled Jeanne Lanvin, Paris, Castillo. An unusual combination of colors that are striking together.

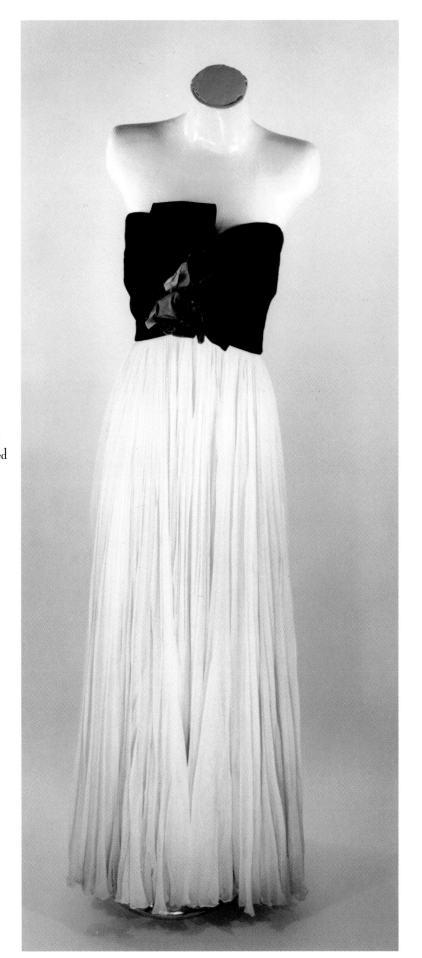

Ca. 1953 strapless evening gown, with a black silk velvet bodice and a white silk chiffon skirt; decorated with a single, burgundy silk velvet rose at the waistline; lined with white silk; labeled Sarmi, New York. An incredibly beautiful gown!

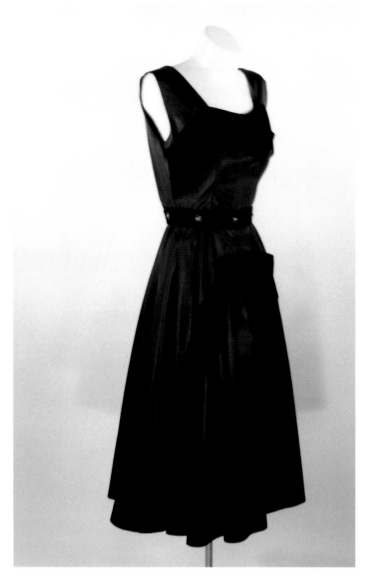

Ca. 1950 black taffeta cocktail dress, trimmed with large, asymmetrical black velvet bows; belt studded with rhinestones.

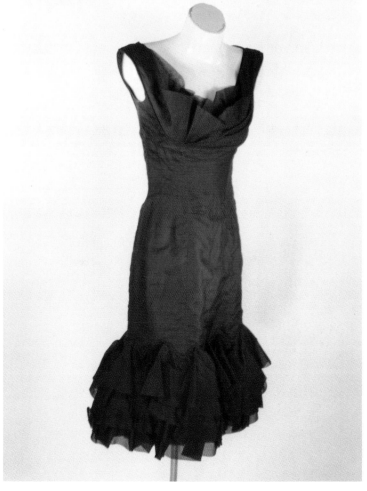

Ca. 1950 black silk cocktail dress; labeled Ceil Chapman. A structurally fascinating dress!

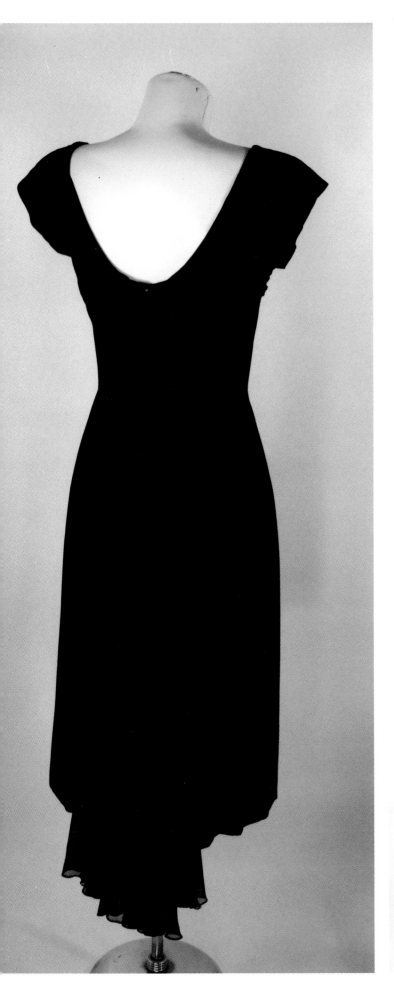

Ca. 1950 black silk and silk chiffon cocktail dress; beige and black silk chiffon used on bodice which continues to back of dress and ties; labeled Bird-Speakman, Inc., Wilmington, Del. (A retailer of high-quality women's clothing).

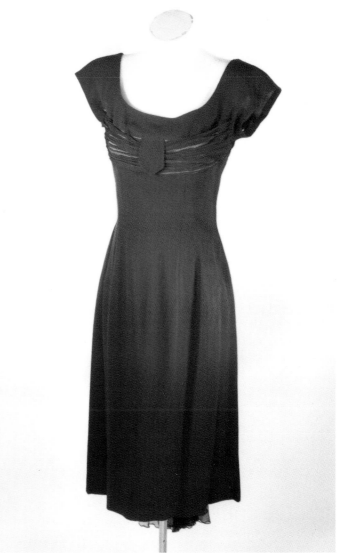

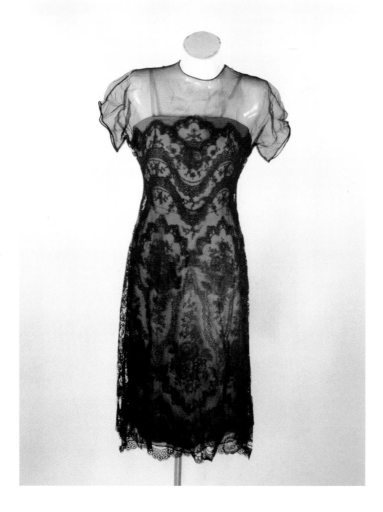

Ca. 1950 black silk lace dress; bodice of silk illusion; underdress of beige silk chiffon over beige silk; labeled Irene, Exclusively For Nan Duskin, Philadelphia.

Ca. 1955 white cotton piqué bustier, with a single strap which is embroidered and decorated with pink straw flowers; fully lined with white batiste; labeled Made in Italy by Fuilio, Capri, Florence.

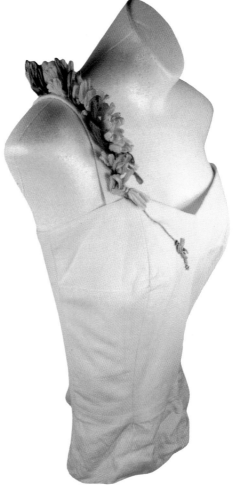

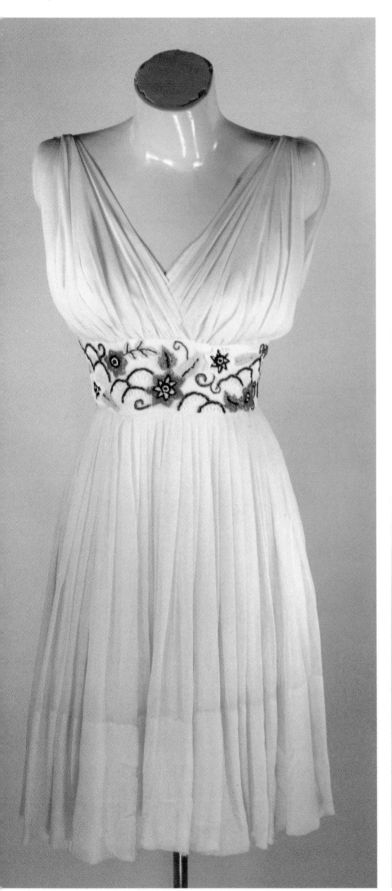

Ca. 1953 white silk chiffon cocktail dress; midriff decorated with round, glass beads in shades of red, black, pale green, and tan; skirt has two layers of silk chiffon; dress is fully lined with white silk; labeled Elissa. A "Marilyn" dress!

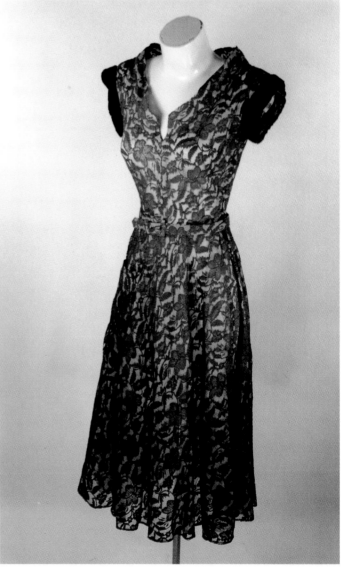

Ca. 1950 blue lace over beige silk chiffon, with a matching belt, and blue silk velvet detailing on the cap sleeves.

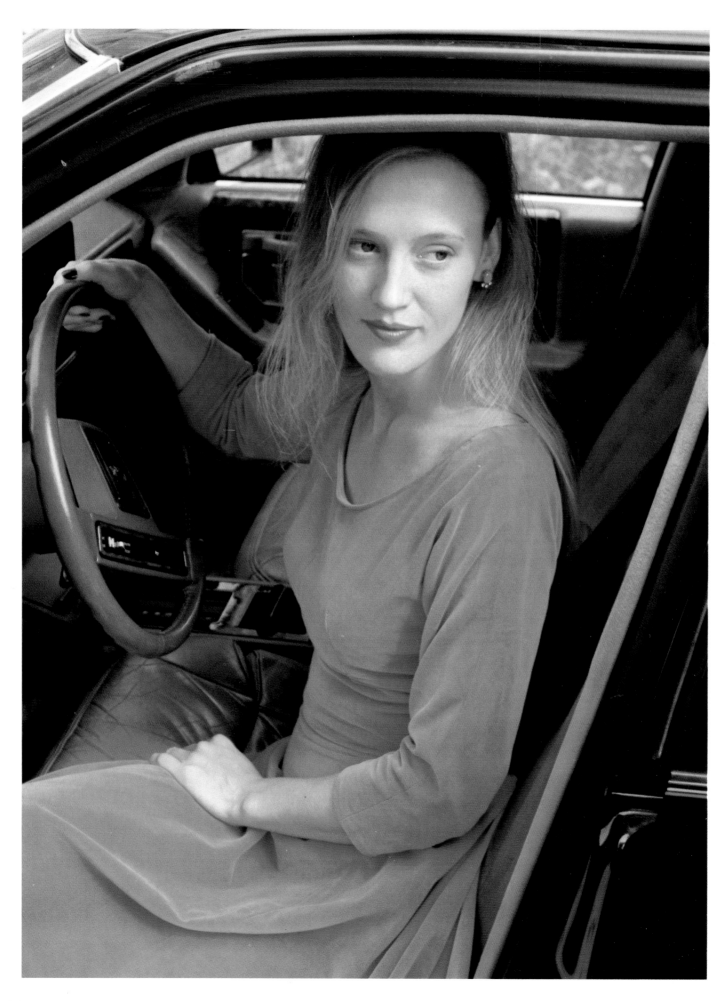

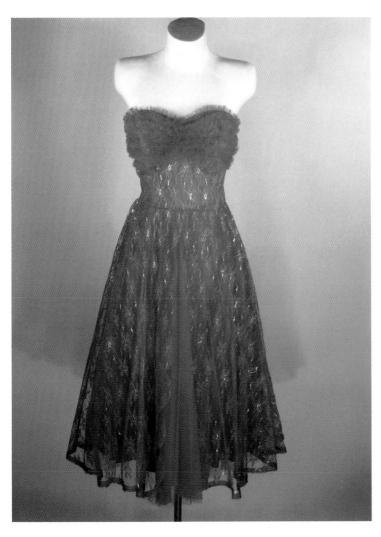

Ca. 1955 red net strapless prom gown; lined with red taffeta; decorated with silver metallic embroidery.

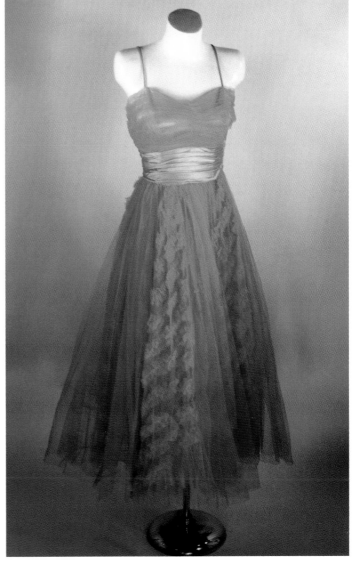

Ca. 1950 rose velveteen princess style dress. *Modeled by Marcie Behanna.*

Ca. 1955 rose net prom gown; taffeta cummerbund waist; "spaghetti" straps; lined with rose taffeta. The typical net prom gown of the 1950s!

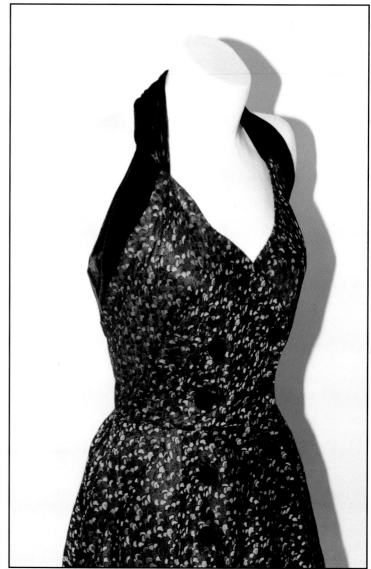

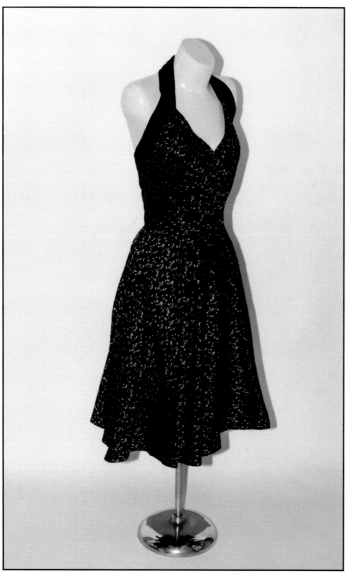

Ca. 1954 black and tan brocade and velvet cocktail dress, with a matching jacket and scarf; elaborate halter-style wrap dress, with black velvet covered buttons; labeled Jacques Fath of Paris-New York, Designs For joseph halpert. Jacques Fath began to design clothes for joseph halpert in the late 1940s.

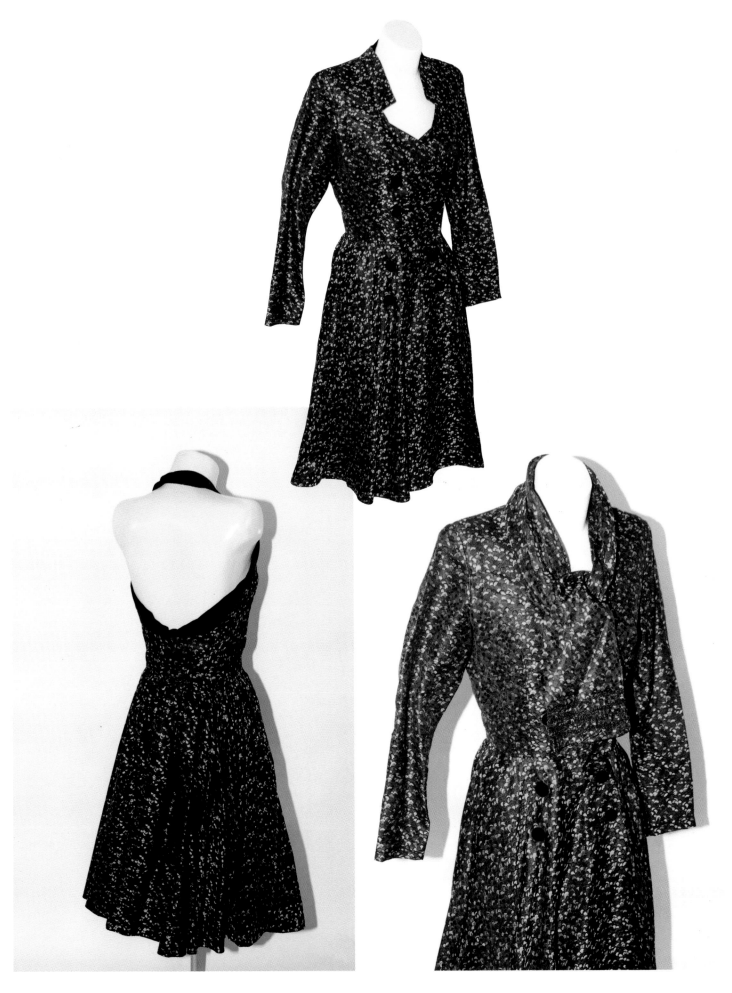

Ca. 1955 red cotton dress, embroidered all over in a white floral pattern; sleeveless, with a circular, gathered skirt; labeled Anne Fogarty, Margot Inc.

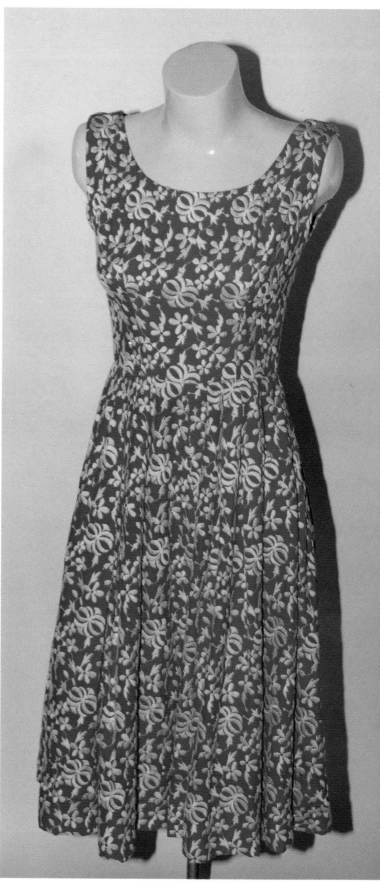

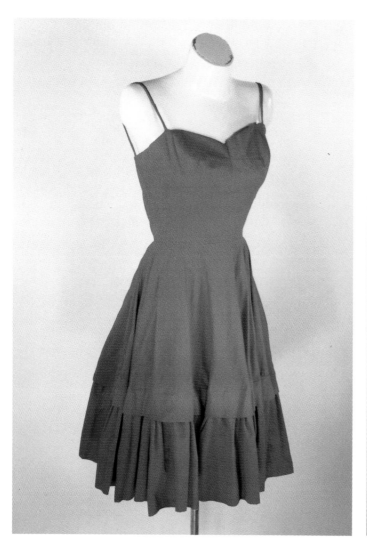

Ca. 1955 red cotton gown; bodice elaborately boned and lined with white cotton; labeled Roselyne Vard, Cannes, 35 La Croisette 36.

Ca. 1955 printed silk dress, with large, "realistic" roses; lined with a lighter-weight version of the same printed silk; labeled Scaasi.

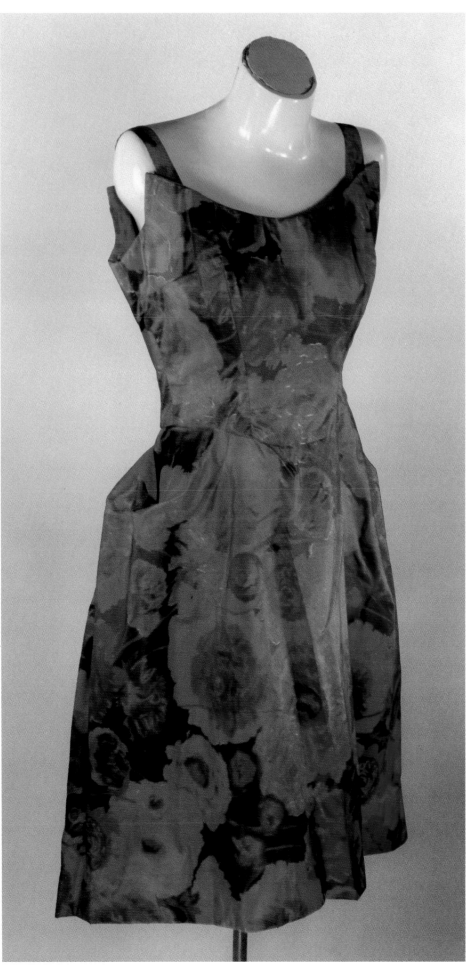

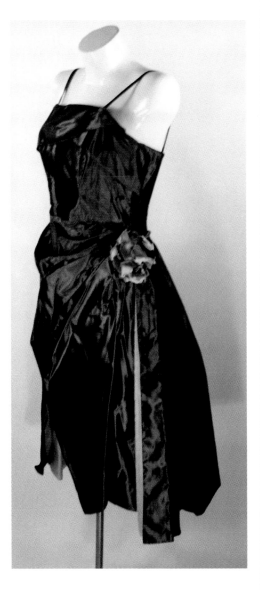

Ca. 1950 rust brown and beige iridescent taffeta cocktail dress, "spaghetti" straps; beige and rust brown silk rose at waist.

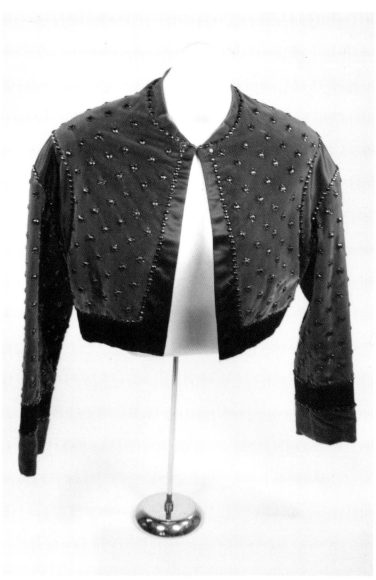

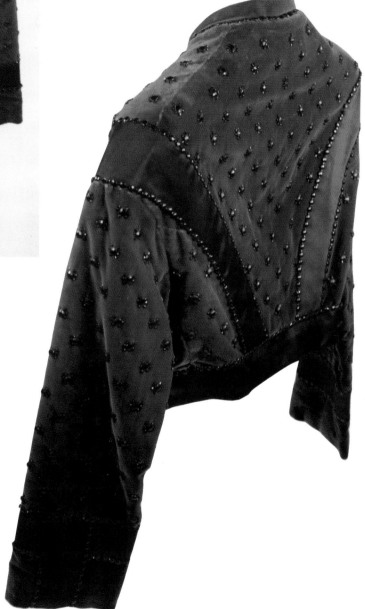

Ca. 1955 brown silk velvet and black silk satin dinner jacket; decorated all over with black glass beads, some in clusters; lined with black silk satin; labeled Bergdorf Goodman.

1960s

Hemlines soon become the issue of the 1960s. Skirts plummet from high-thigh to ankle length and anything goes! Unconventional designs gain wide acceptance--the British invasion, Mary Quant, granny boots, "mod" styles, floral prints and "flower power." Perhaps because of America's obsession with Jacqueline Kennedy, there is a heightened awareness of couture clothing. An eclectic decade in fashion, the 1960s is probably best known for the demise of millinery.

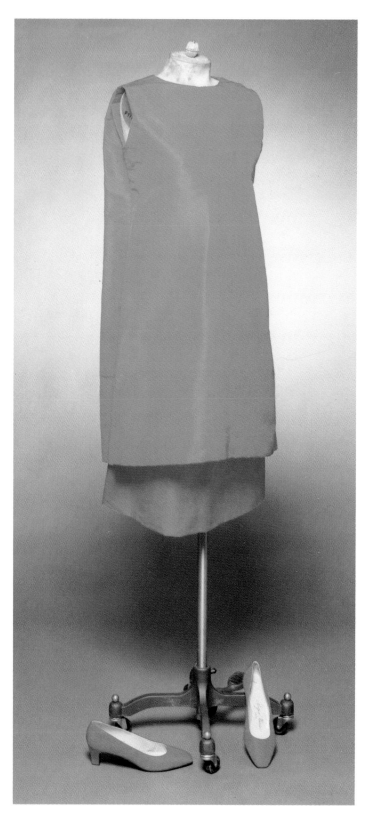

Ca. 1960 red silk taffeta dress with a shiny, reflective surface and "leopard spotted" markings; labeled Givenchy. Shoes by Roger Vivier. *Courtesy of Mark Walsh. Photograph by Kelly Wright.*

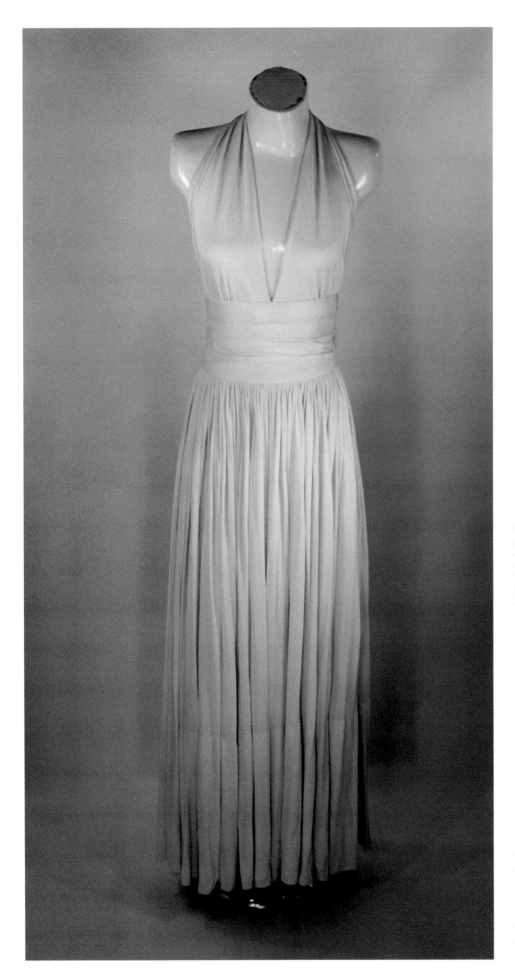

Ca. 1960 ivory silk jersey halter-style evening gown; lined with white silk crepe; labeled Norman Norell, New York. Incredible simplicity and elegance—a truly beautiful gown!

Ca. 1960 pale gray silk chiffon gown, embroidered with silver metallic thread and elaborately decorated all over with rhinestones, many of which are "dangling;" trimmed with white mink; lined with pale gray silk; labeled Sarmi, New York.

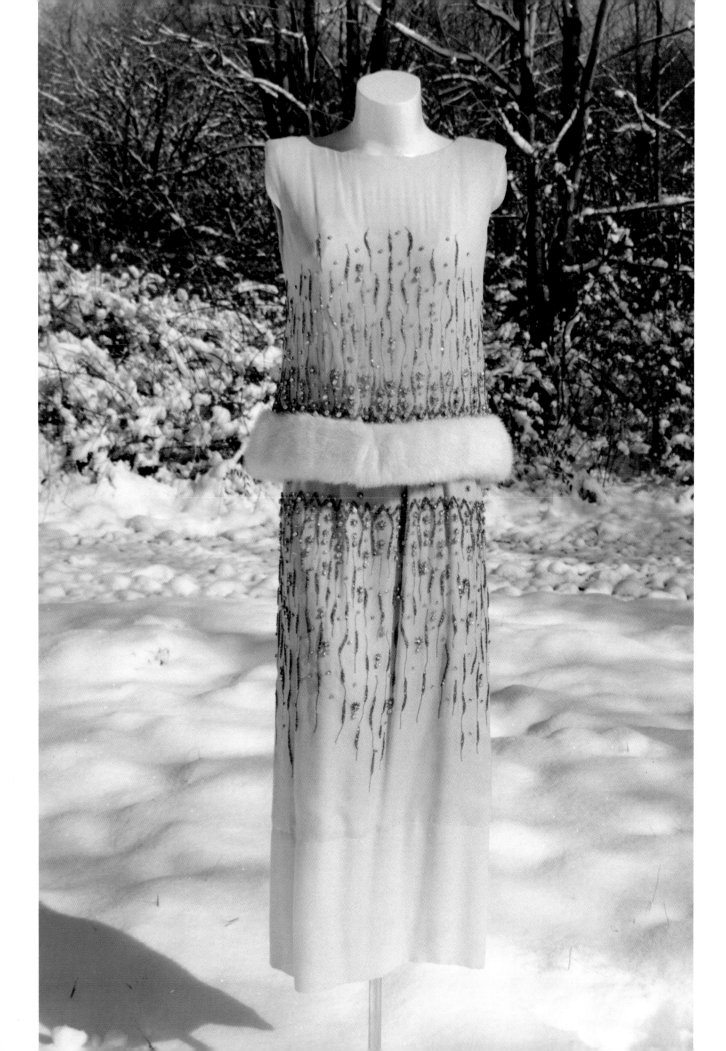

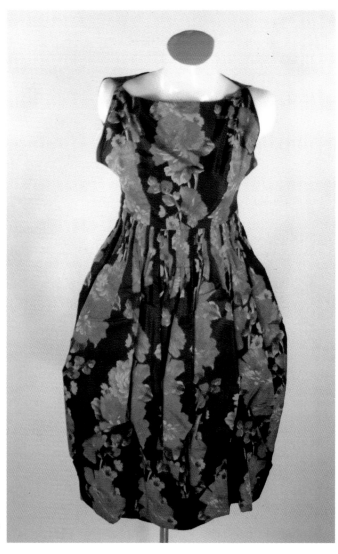

Ca. 1960 cocktail dress; black silk with red roses; elaborately gathered and draped skirt; labeled Galanos.

Matching coat with wide belt; lined with lightweight silk in the same print; labeled Galanos.

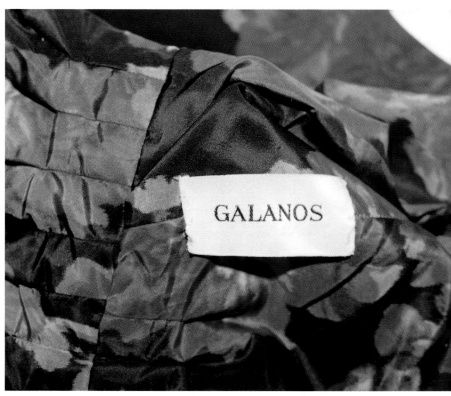

Ca. 1960 black silk lace cocktail dress, decorated with large, black sequins, and round, black glass beads; strapless underdress of beige silk; matching jacket, not shown.

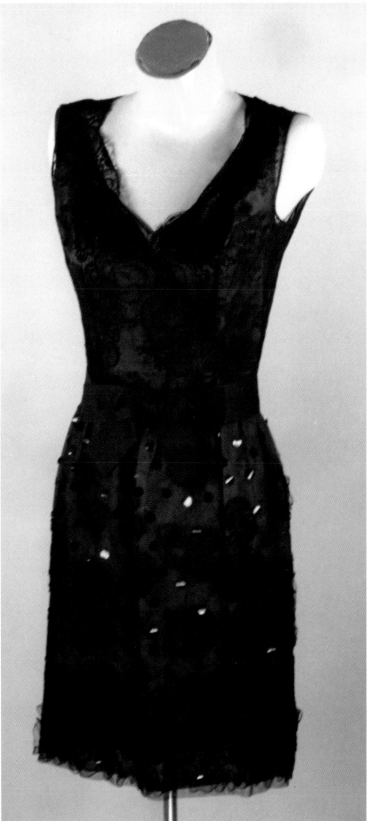

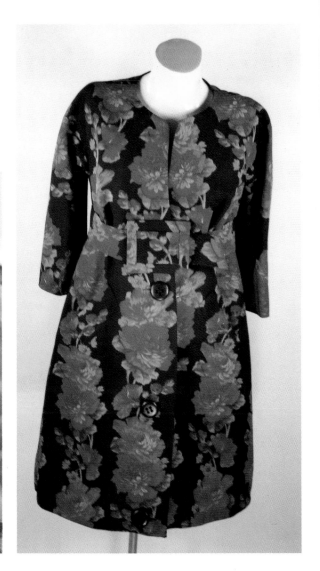

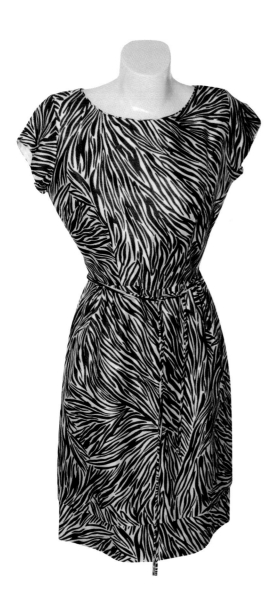

Ca. 1960 black and white silk printed dress, with a layered skirt; lined with white taffeta.

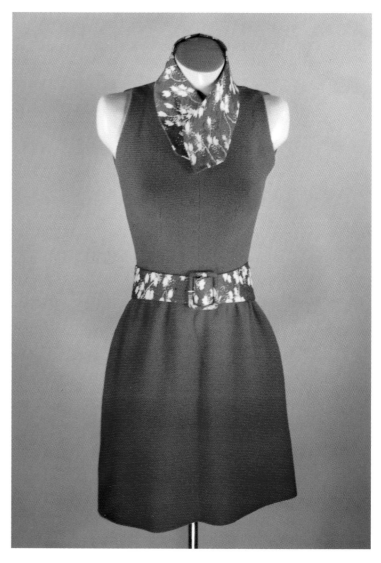

Ca. 1965 burnt-orange wool knit dress; kidskin lined cotton brocade belt and matching scarf; matching wool knit large shawl (not pictured); labeled pauline trigere.

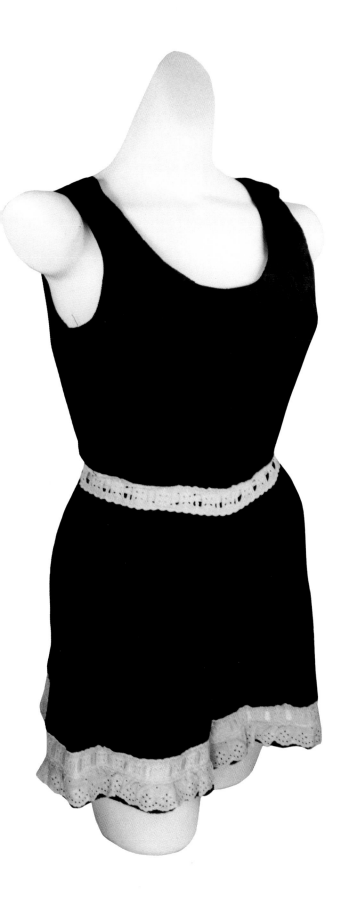

Ca. 1965 black silk velvet "romper," (short pants and attached bodice), trimmed at the waist and shorts' bottoms with white eyelet and ribbon; labeled Mary Quant's ginger Group, Made In England, Showcase 5 Gimbels. These were clearly before "hot pants," which did not become fashionable until the early 1970s.

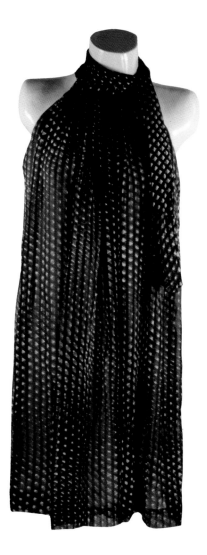

Ca. 1965 printed silk chiffon dress, in shades of brown and tan; lined with tan silk crepe; labeled pauline trigere.

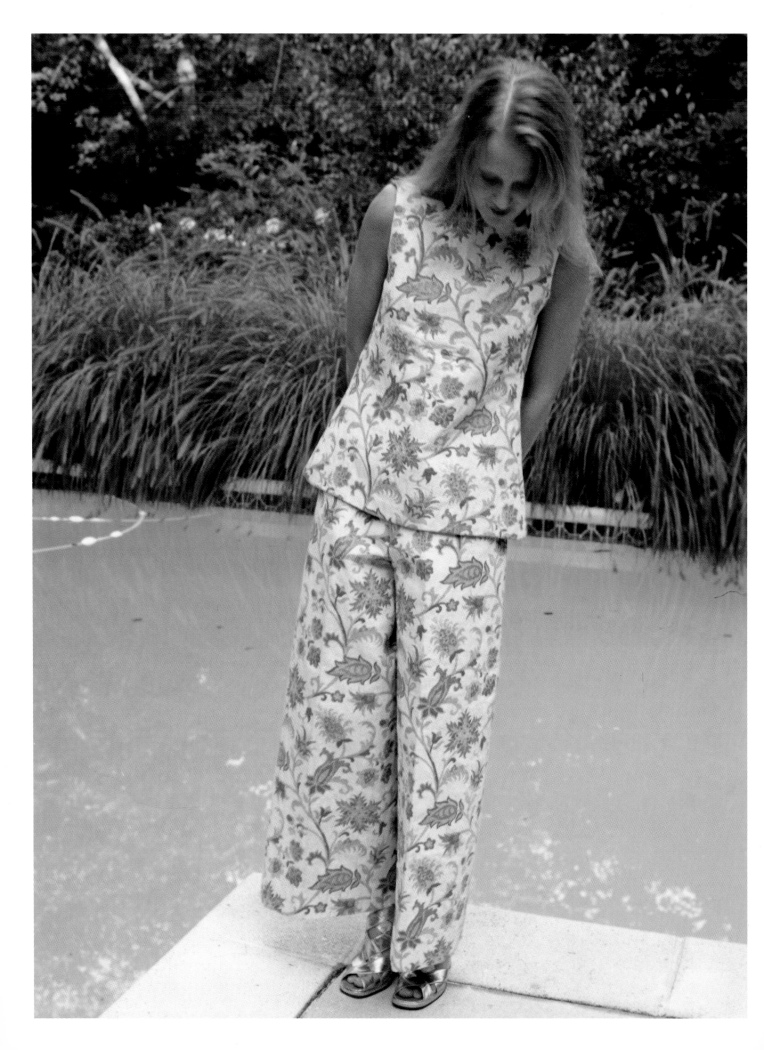

Chapter 2
Couture

Couture is a French term used throughout the fashion industry to describe the original styles, the ultimate in fine sewing and tailoring, the finest and most expensive fabrics. The term *haute couture* (oht kootoor) derives from the French meaning "highest quality dressmaking" and applies to the top designers of custom-made clothes. Couture designs are shown publicly in *collections* twice a year--spring/summer and fall/winter.

It gets more complex considering the roles of the organizations formed to promote the fashion. *Fairchild's Dictionary of Fashion* defines the purposes of several of these important organizations. *Chambre Syndicale de la Couture Parisienne* was founded in 1868 by Parisian couturiers, the most influential of whom was Charles Frederick Worth. An outgrowth of medieval guilds, it regulates its members concerning piracy of styles, dates of openings for collections, number of models presented, relations with the press, questions relating to law and taxes, and promotional activities. In 1970, some "ready-to-wear" firms were permitted membership. The school sponsored by the association was organized in 1930, and is called *l'Escole de la Chambre Syndicale de la Couture*. Similar organizations exist for milliners (*Chambre Syndicale de la Mode*) and for accessory houses (*Chambre Syndicale des Paruriers*). Another vehicle for promotion was formed in 1975, (*Chambre Syndicale du Prêt-à-Porter, des Couturiers et Createurs de Mode),* which includes couture and "ready-to-wear" designers.

The concept of "ready-to-wear" clothes derives from the French term prêt-à-porter, which translates as "ready to be carried." In other words, the clothes we think of as "off-the-rack" or "ready-to-wear" are those clothes that are already made, as opposed to clothes that must be custom-made, or made-to-order.. Long before the industrial revolution, such clothes were available, but it took the industrial revolution to put large numbers on the racks and shelves, in general stores, speciality stores, and department stores. Clothing was being mass-produced before 1900. *The International Ladies' Garment Workers' Union*, a semi-industrial union of U. S. and Canadian needle-trades workers, was founded in 1900 to provide services for its members and to fight against poor working conditions and unfair labor practices. "Sizing" made it possible to cut garments to fit a variety of body types, making "ready-to-wear" more affordable. Even if the most expensive fabrics are used in "ready-to-wear," the individual piece costs less because there is no time spent in "fitting," the trade term for the dressmaker's or tailor's session with the customer for altering the garment to fit the customer.

Ca. 1965 brocade pants suit, in shades of ivory, beige, and copper; silk lined; back zipper; worn with period appropriate gold platform sandals; labeled a junior sophisticates original, Bonwit Teller. *Modeled by Marcie Behanna.*

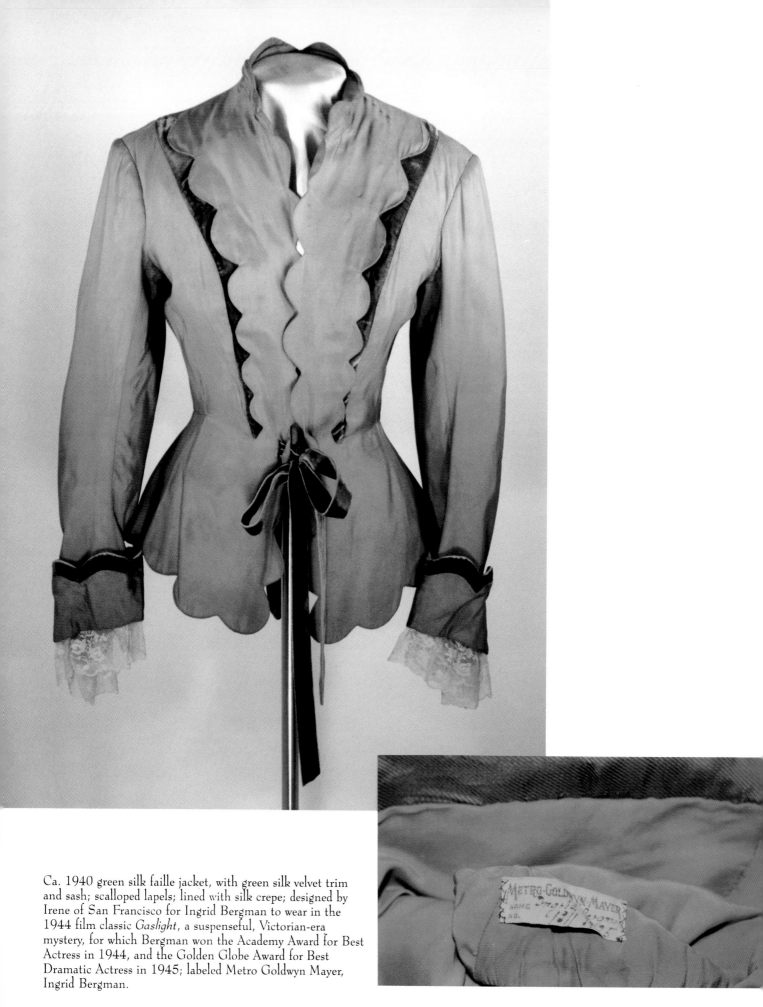

Ca. 1940 green silk faille jacket, with green silk velvet trim and sash; scalloped lapels; lined with silk crepe; designed by Irene of San Francisco for Ingrid Bergman to wear in the 1944 film classic *Gaslight*, a suspenseful, Victorian-era mystery, for which Bergman won the Academy Award for Best Actress in 1944, and the Golden Globe Award for Best Dramatic Actress in 1945; labeled Metro Goldwyn Mayer, Ingrid Bergman.

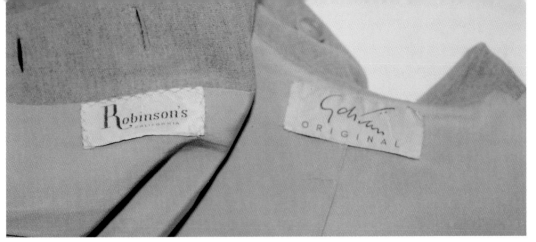

Ca. 1945 mustard color, lightweight, wool tweed jacket, inset with same material design, front and back; lined with crepe; labeled Adrian Original, Robinson's, California. An exceptionally beautifully, tailored jacket. *Courtesy of the Drexel Historic Costume Collection.*

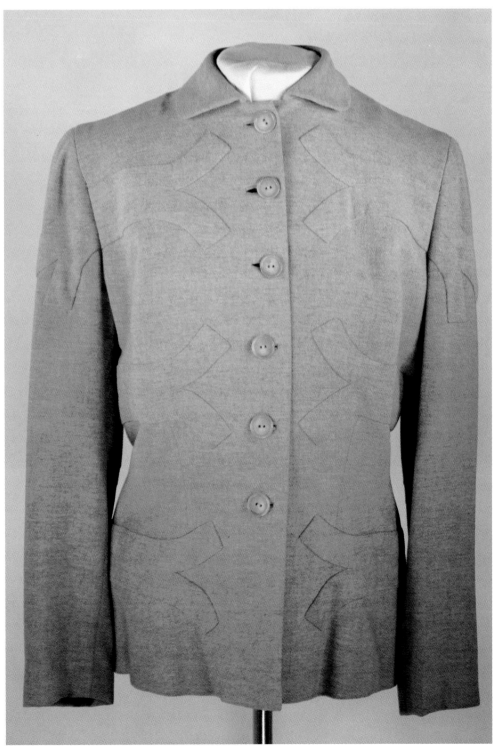

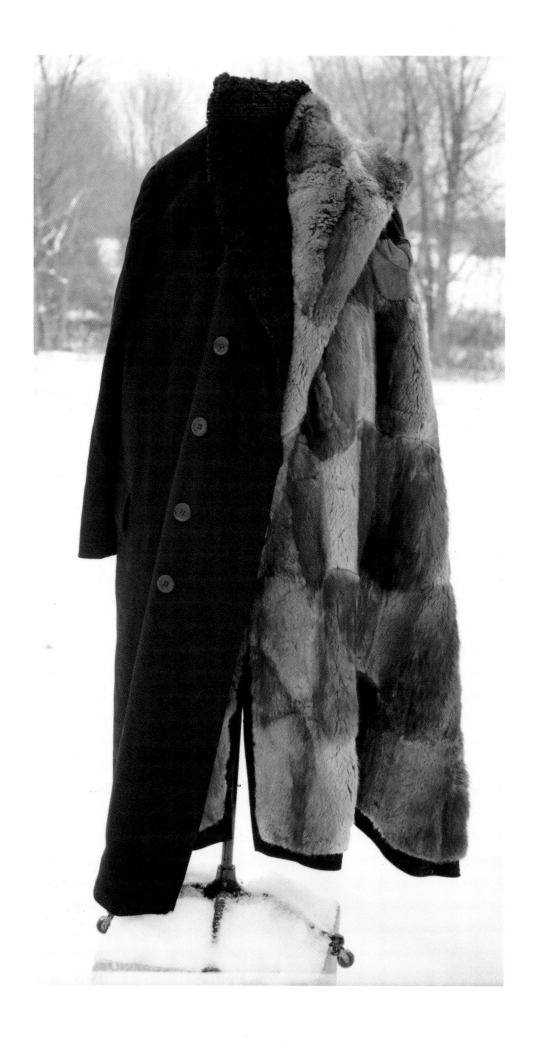

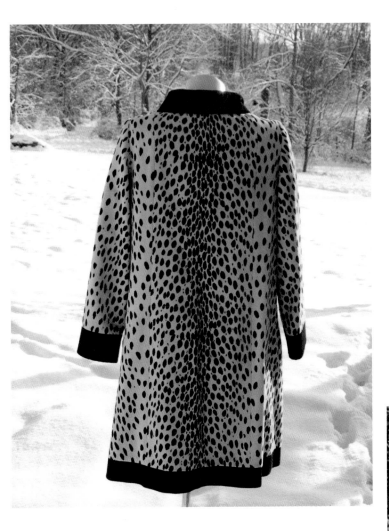

Ca. 1964 ivory and black velvet "spotted" coat, as viewed from the back; labeled Funny Girl Trade Mark, c.R.S. '64, Cathy Dee.

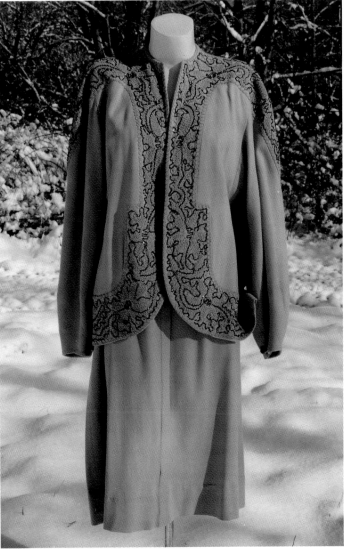

Ca. 1940 pale gray wool challis suit, decorated in same-color soutache and charcoal gray round, glass beads; jacket lined with tan crepe; labeled Evalen Original, New York.

Ca. 1920 man's, double-breasted, black wool coat, with a black Persian lamb collar; lined with beaver; underarms lined in tan leather.

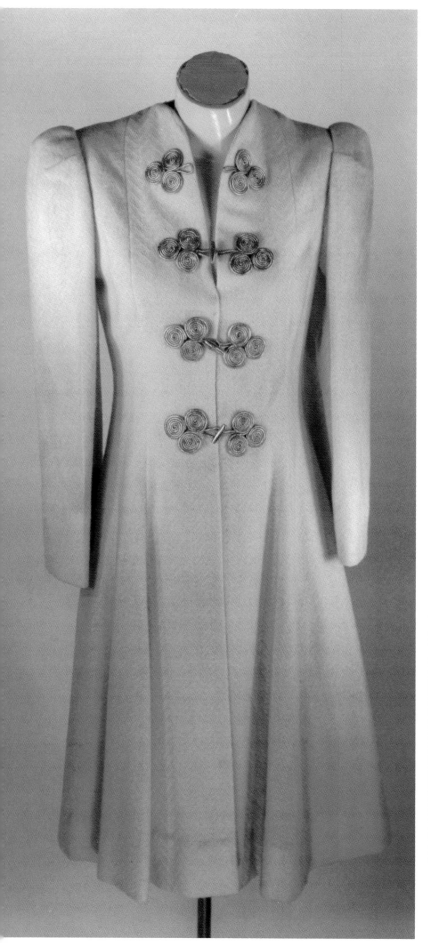

Ca. 1930 white wool coat,
fastened with gold frogs; lined with
taffeta.

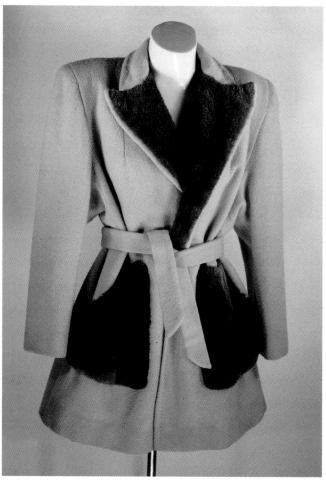

Ca. 1940 yellow cashmere coat,
trimmed with beaver; lined with
yellow silk crepe; labeled Bonwit
Teller.

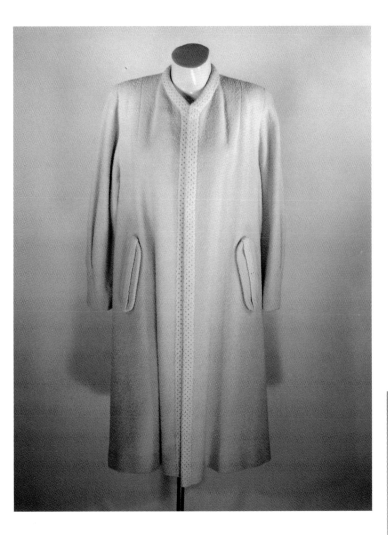

Ca. 1950 ivory wool wrap coat, trimmed with ivory and tan tweed; taffeta lined; labeled Anglo Fabrics, 100% Wool.

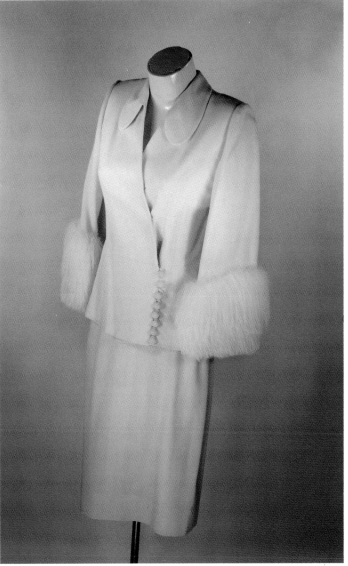

Ca. 1955 white wool challis suit, with fur-trimmed sleeves; wrap-style jacket with eight covered buttons; entirely lined with white silk crepe; labeled Lilli Ann of San Francisco. *Courtesy of Lois Fischer.*

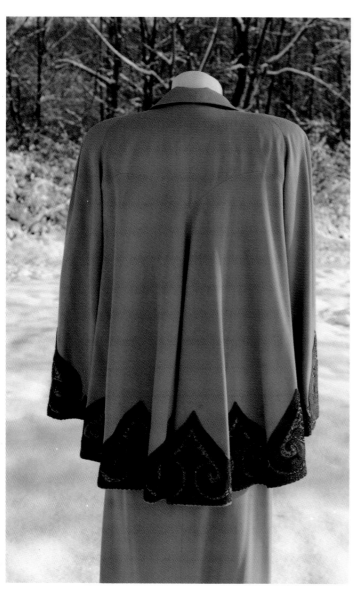

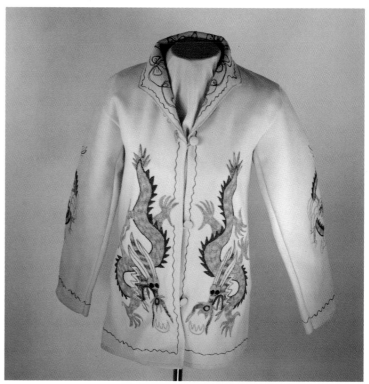

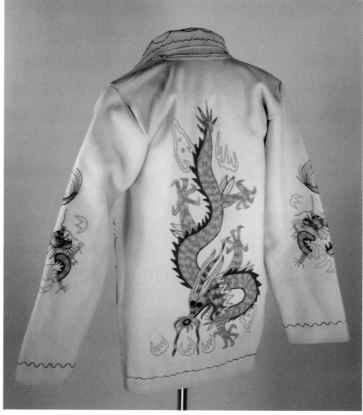

Ca. 1940 tan wool gabardine suit, decorated with brown soutache and bugle beads; swing style jacket with straight skirt; jacket lined with tan silk crepe; labeled Jean's, Providence, Forstmann, 100% Virgin Wool.

Ca. 1950 ivory wool flannel jacket, embroidered with orange and green dragons on the back, front, and sleeves. This is a most unusual Oriental jacket.

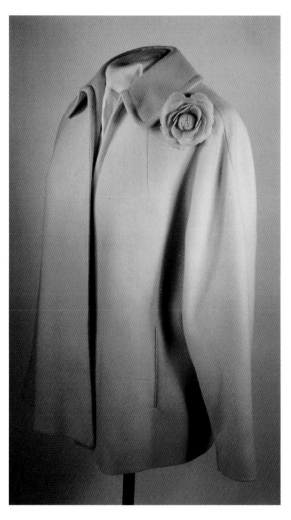

Ca. 1950 warm beige wrap jacket, decorated with a single rose of the same material; lined with ivory crepe.

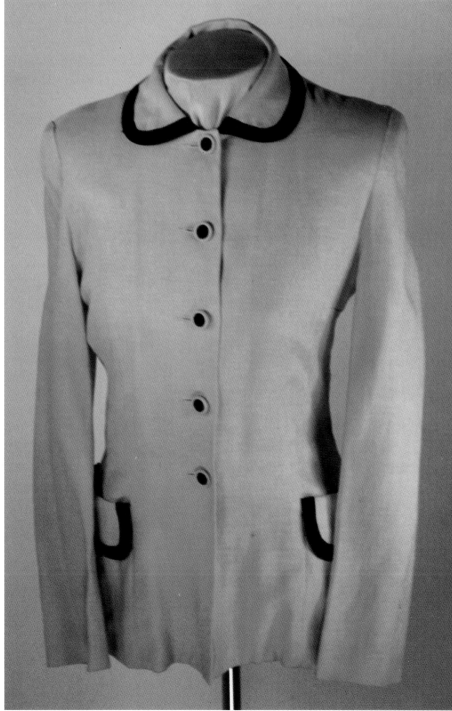

Ca. 1940 beige linen jacket, trimmed with navy blue; covered buttons; unlined.

Ca. 1940 plaid wool jacket, in shades of brown, tan, and light green; Bakelite buttons; lined with tan crepe.

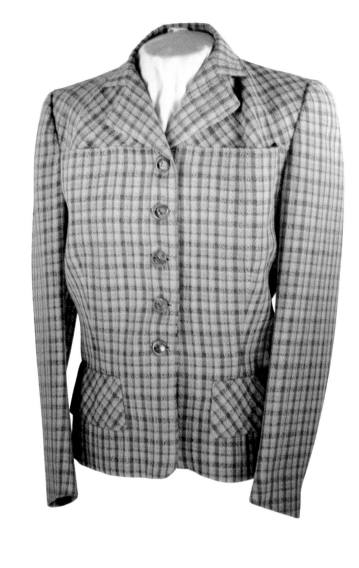

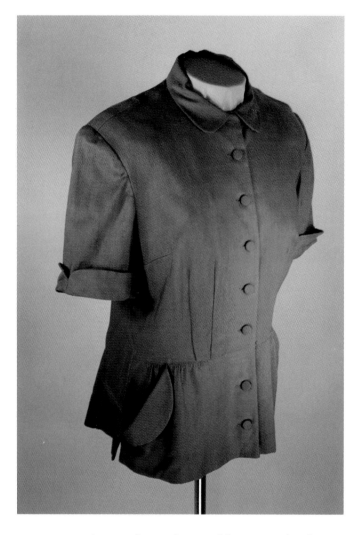

Ca. 1950 tan linen jacket, with covered buttons; unlined.

Ca. 1940 beige and tan plaid tweed jacket, with a collar-scarf of orange velvet; wooden buttons; lined with tan crepe.

Ca. 1940 plaid tweed suit in shades of gray, tan, and pale yellow; Bakelite buttons; jacket lined with tan crepe; labeled The Lortay, Made Expressly for Lord & Taylor.

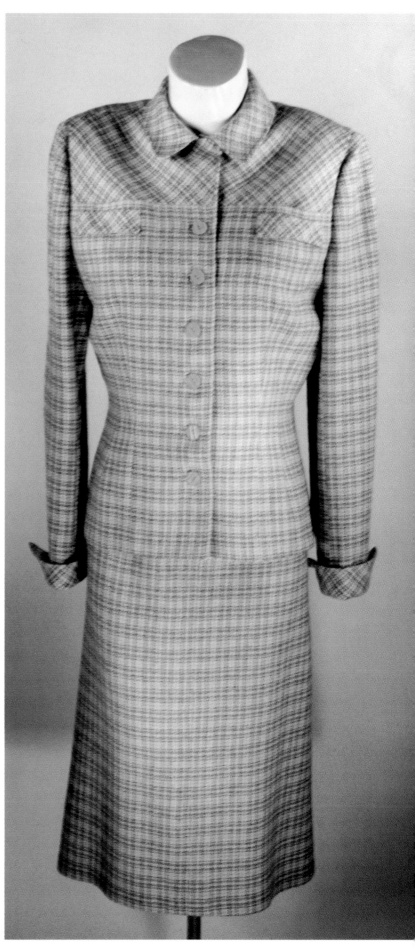

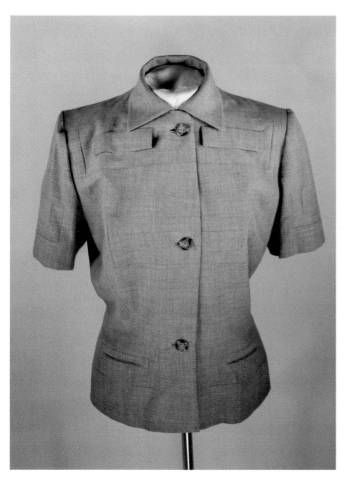

Ca. 1945 gray wool gabardine jacket, with short sleeves; labeled Adrian Original. *Courtesy of the Drexel Historic Costume Collection.*

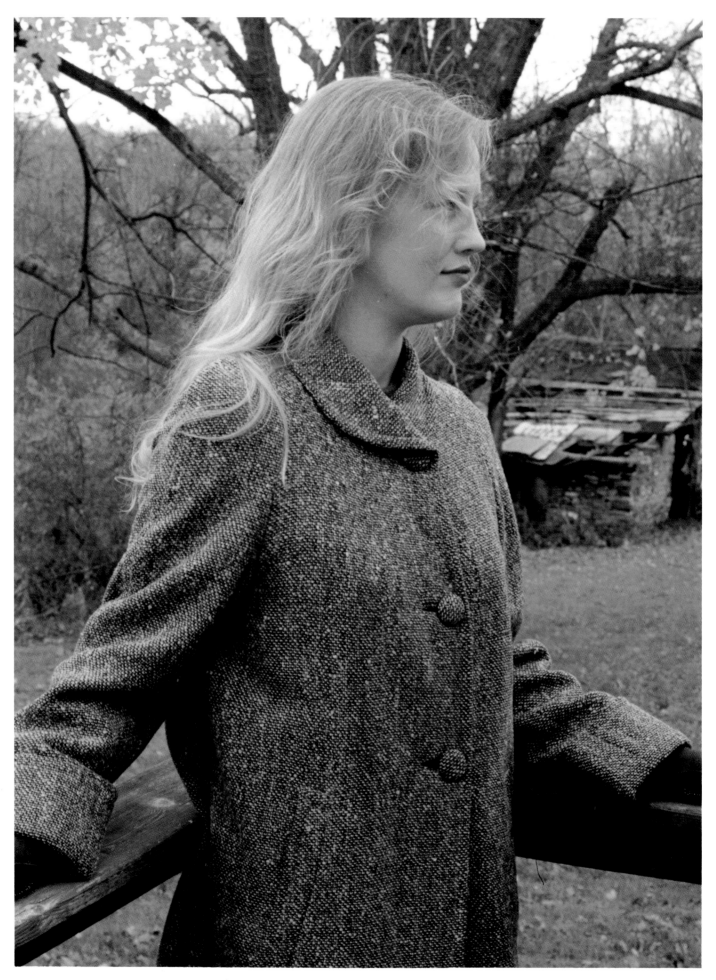

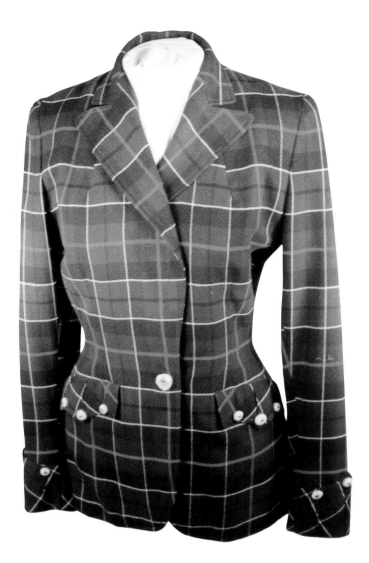

Ca. 1935 blue, green, and red plaid jacket with carved bone buttons; lined with navy blue crepe; labeled Joseph de V. Keefe, Haverford, Pa.

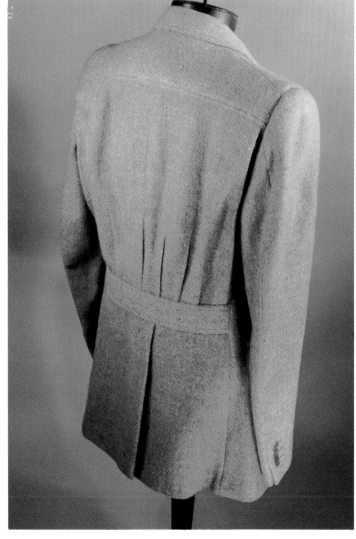

Ca. 1945 blue, orange, and brown tweed coat; single breasted with two buttons on each wide cuff; lined with tan crepe; labeled Tailored by hope, Souderton, PA. *Modeled by Marcie Behanna.*

Ca. 1935 man's tan tweed suit jacket, shown from the back; lined with brown silk; labeled inside the matching vest, Michael A. Rienzi & Company, Incorporated, Mr. C. Brewster Rhoads, Date 10-25-35, No. 6912; labeled additionally in the suit jacket, Rienzi, Philadelphia. A beautifully tailored jacket showing detailing typical of the period.

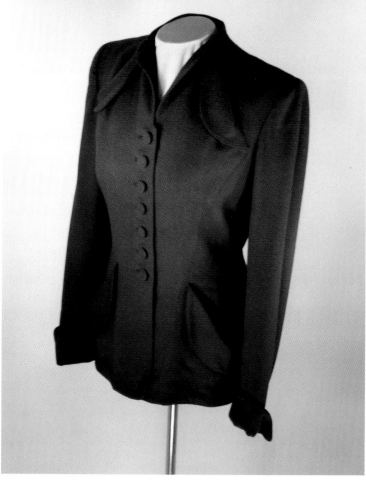

Ca. 1945 burgundy cashmere jacket; covered and embroidered buttons; lined with silk satin; labeled Emil E. Otto, Allentown, Lancaster.

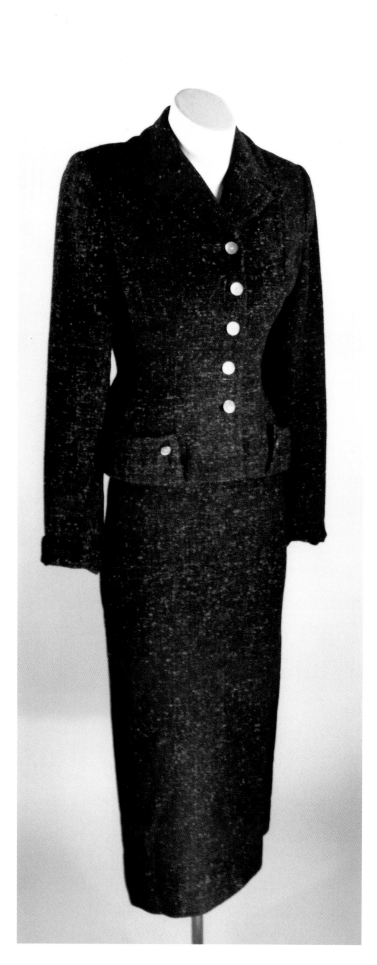

Ca. 1945 burgundy tweed suit, with mother-of-pearl buttons; jacket lined with burgundy iridescent taffeta; labeled Fashioned and Tailored by Laura Dale Jr., New York,

Ca. 1940 navy blue wool gabardine suit; decorated with six glass buttons, and two "working buttons" at the collar; belted; lined with blue crepe. A very unusual jacket!

Ca. 1940 blue and white houndstooth tweed suit; jacket lined with blue crepe. Great button detailing!

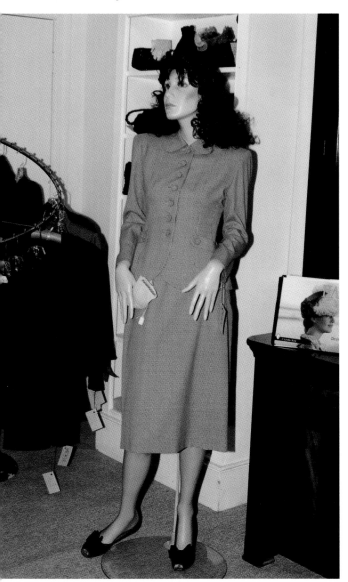

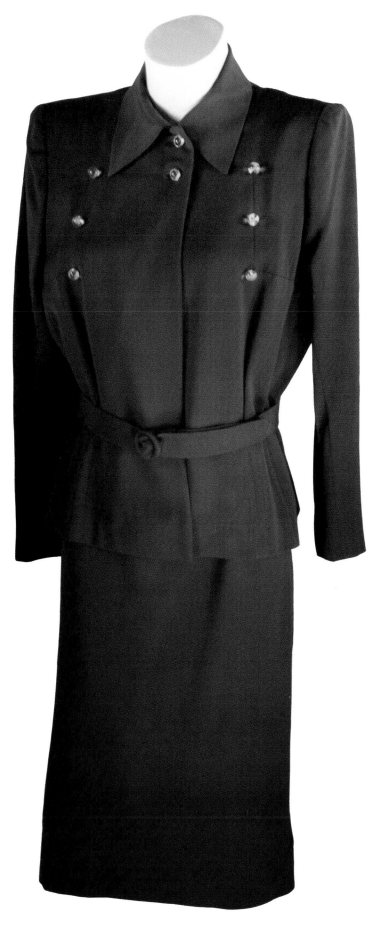

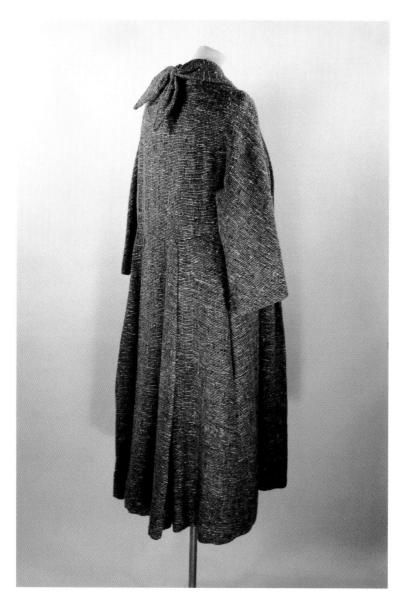

Ca. 1950 brown, tan, and red tweed wrap coat, with pleats from the waist down, and a collar that "ties" in back; lined with copper silk taffeta.

Ca. 1950 dark rose wool challis coat, lined with navy blue silk crepe; labeled Eisenberg Originals. A structurally fascinating coat, with great wide cuffs! *Modeled by Marcie Behanna.*

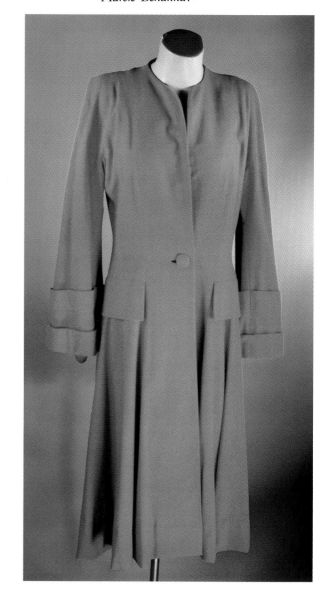

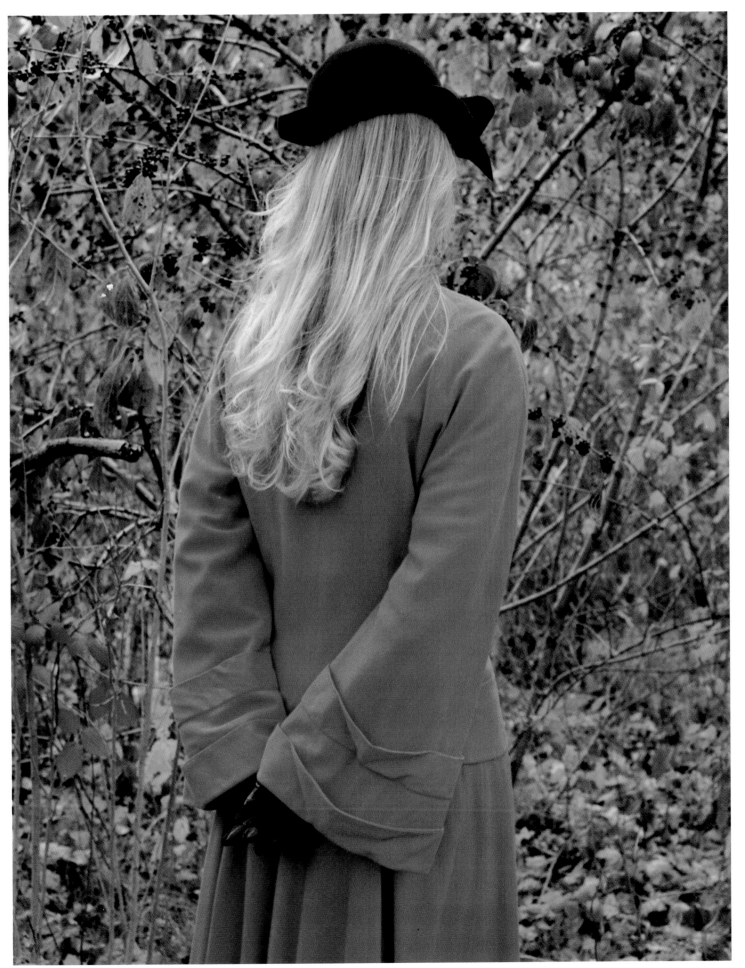

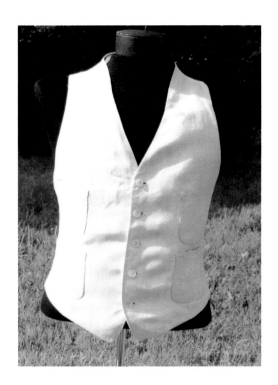

Ca. 1920 man's white linen vest. Linen is the fabric of summer, unlike any other!

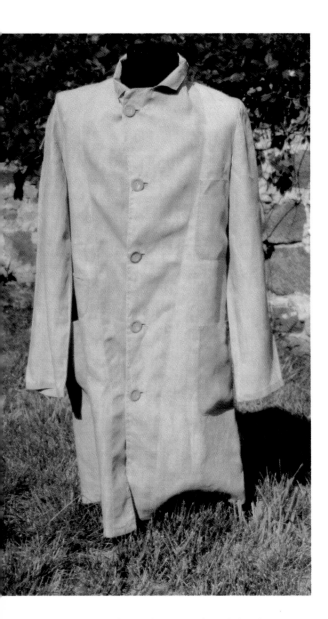

Ca. 1920 tan linen duster, with Bakelite buttons.

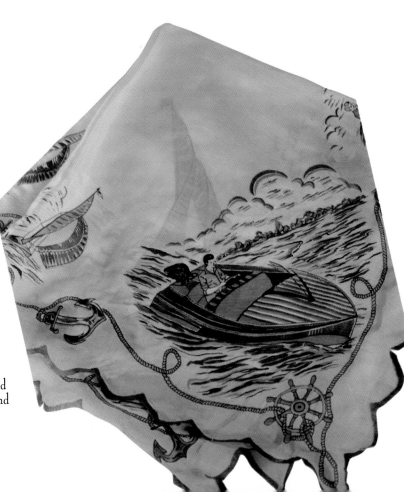

Ca. 1940 yellow silk scarf, printed with boating images, a sailboat and a motor boat; anchors and compasses.

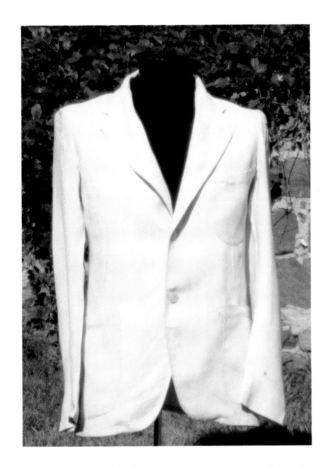

Ca. 1920 man's white linen jacket; unlined; mother-of-pearl buttons.

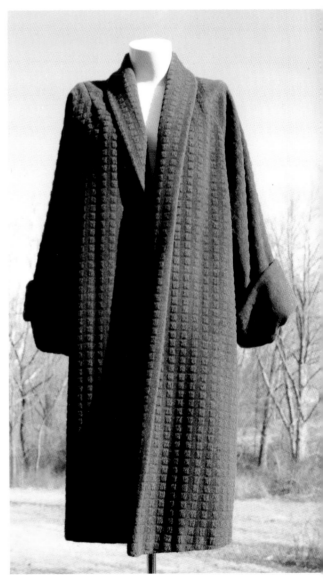

Ca. 1945 plush green wool wrap coat; lined with silk satin; labeled Lilli Ann, San Francisco.

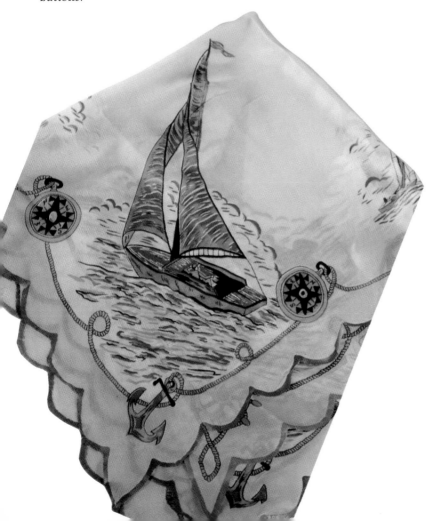

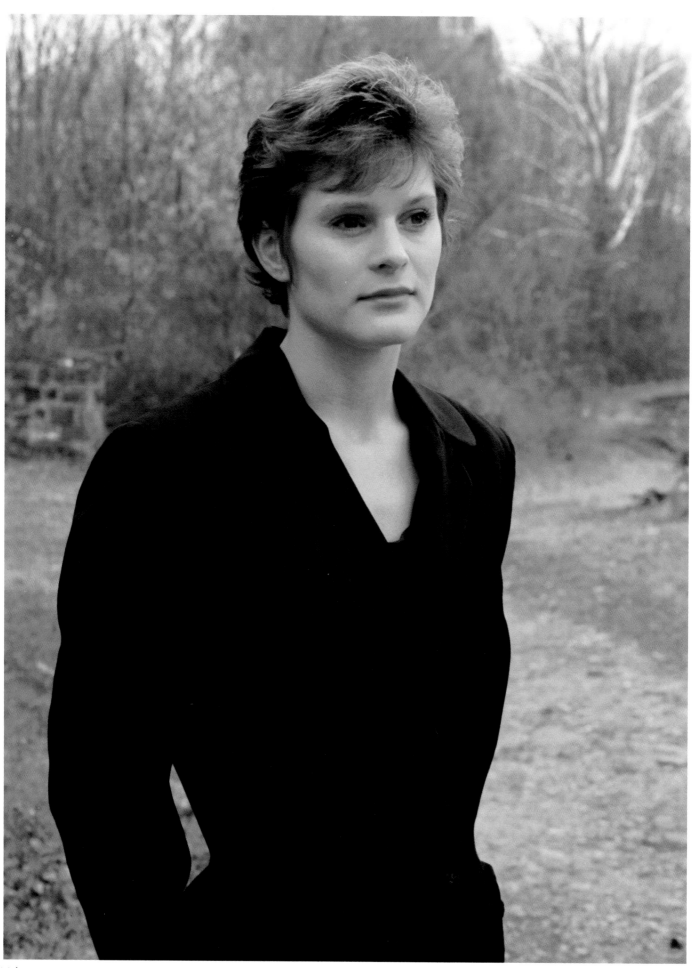

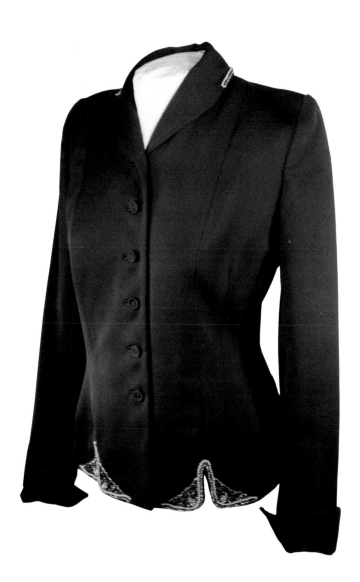

Ca. 1945 gray gabardine jacket, decorated with blue and silver round, glass beads; lined with gray crepe.

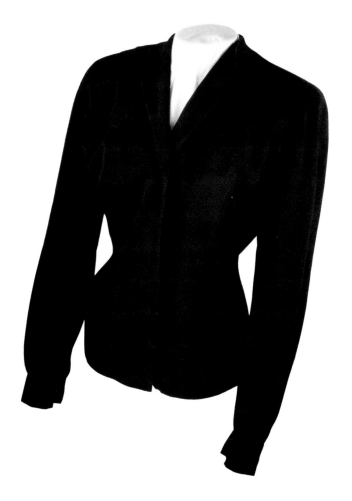

Ca. 1940 navy blue wool gabardine jacket, with covered and embroidered buttons; lined with navy blue crepe; labeled Kaybrooke, New York. *Modeled by Kim Hemingway.*

Ca. 1940 black wool gabardine jacket, with same material inset details on bodice; one covered and embroidered button; full sleeves with two covered and embroidered buttons on each cuff; labeled The Addis Co., Syracuse, New York, Original Bellciano, New York.

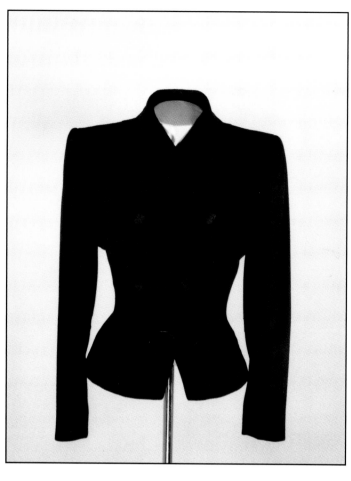

Ca. 1945 black cashmere and wool jacket with unusual woven silk "barrel" buttons, lined with black crepe.

Ca. 1940 burgundy wool ankle length coat; collar decorated all over with diminutive burgundy sequins in a "shooting star" motif; lined with burgundy silk. An incredibly luxurious and beautifully tailored coat! *Modeled by Kim Hemingway.*

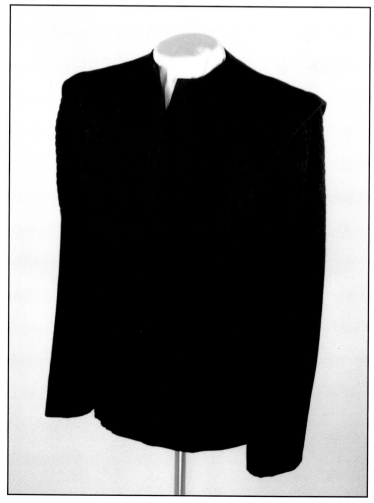

Ca. 1940 black wool flannel jacket, with smocking at the tops of each sleeve; no buttons; labeled Henri Bendel, New York. A beautifully tailored jacket with large shoulder pads.

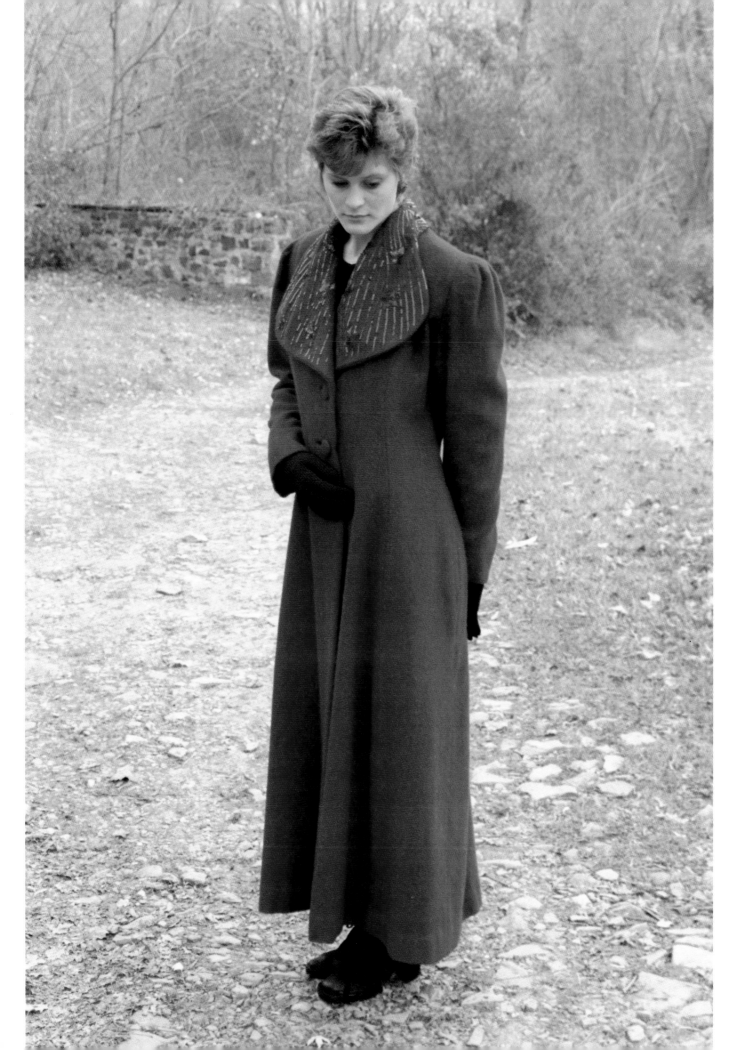

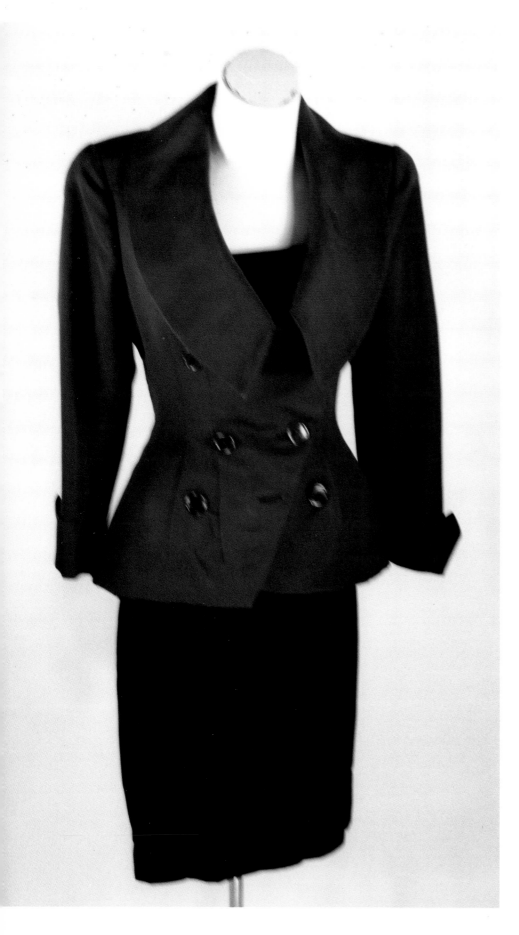

Ca. 1950, black silk faille and velvet suit; silk velvet trim under collar, and skirt is silk velvet; double-breasted jacket with padded hips and one button that is designed with a false button hole; lined with silk satin; labeled Christian Dior-New York Original Trade Mark. This is a structurally beautiful suit, almost architectural in its form.

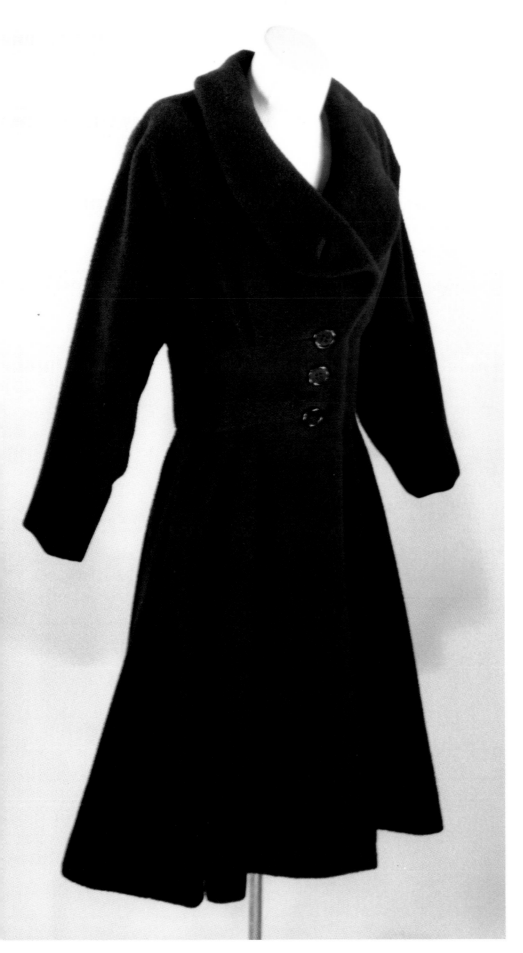

Ca. 1955 black wool princess style coat; lined with black silk; labeled Traina Norell.

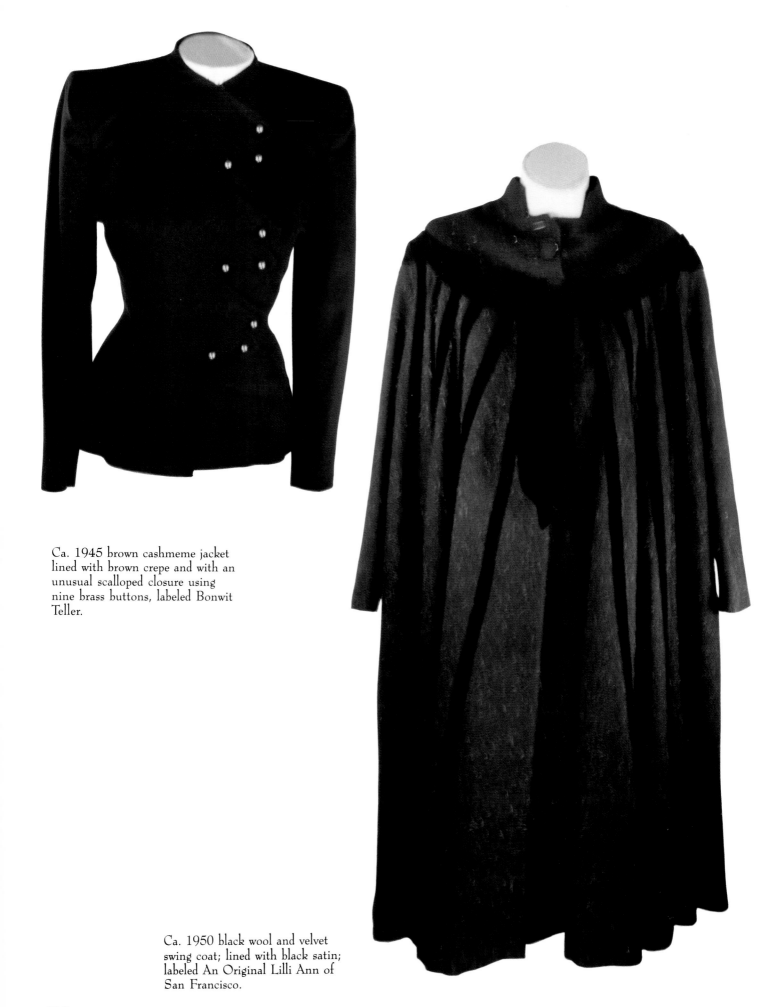

Ca. 1945 brown cashmeme jacket
lined with brown crepe and with an
unusual scalloped closure using
nine brass buttons, labeled Bonwit
Teller.

Ca. 1950 black wool and velvet
swing coat; lined with black satin;
labeled An Original Lilli Ann of
San Francisco.

112

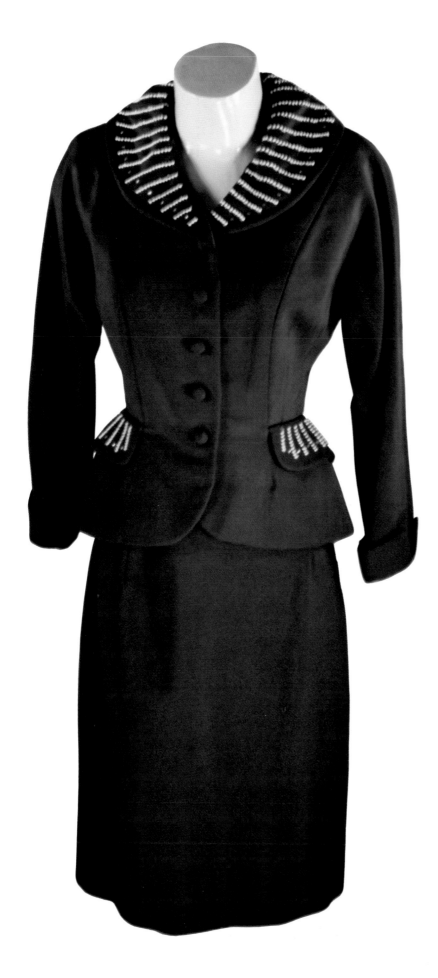

Ca. 1950 gray silk and wool suit, decorated with white beads and rhinestones; covered buttons; jacket lined with white silk crepe; labeled Hollywood, Wilkes Barre, Pa., dan millstein, New York.

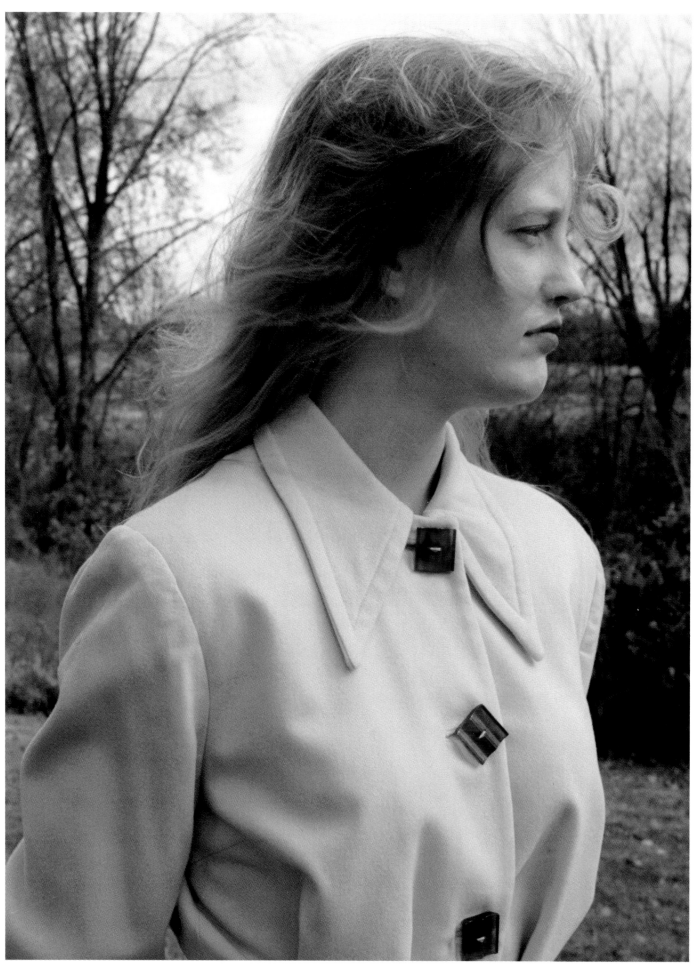

Ca. 1940 pale yellow cashmere jacket, with square Bakelite buttons, and a tie belt. *Modeled by Marcie Behanna.*

Ca. 1920 tan suede gloves, decorated with lighter tan suede diamond patterns.

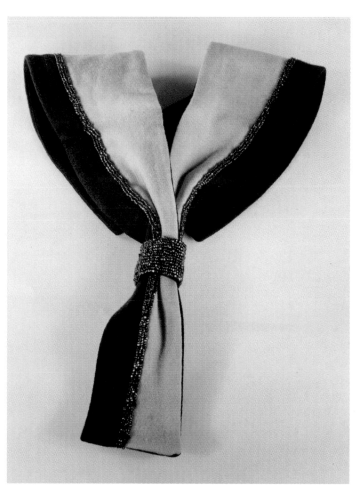

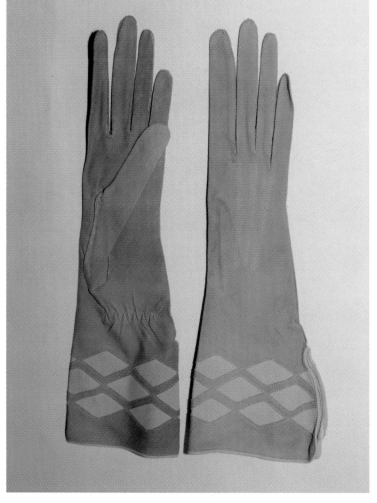

Ca. 1940 collar and tie in shades of tan and brown wool jersey, decorated with copper bugle beads.

Ca. 1965 wide suede belt, with a large, plastic buckle.

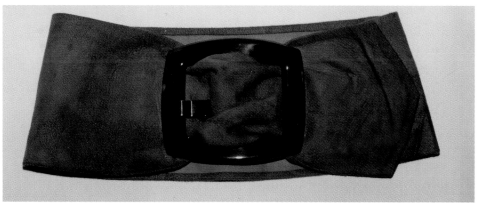

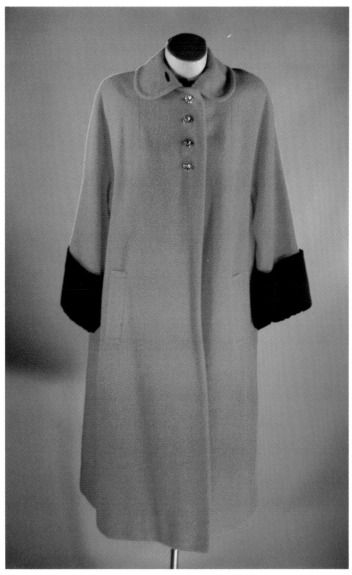

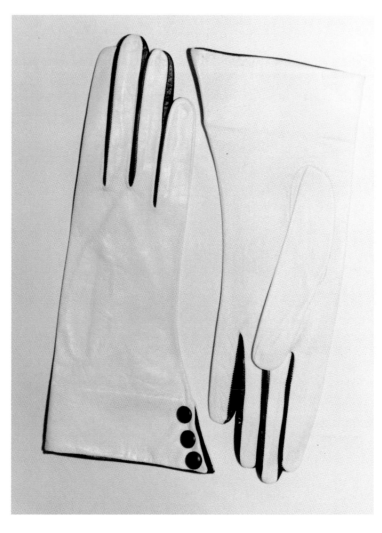

Ca. 1945 white and black kidskin gloves.

Ca. 1950 red wool and cashmere coat, with navy blue wool gabardine cuffs, and glass buttons, surrounded with rhinestones; lined with navy blue and red striped crepe; labeled Tailored by Grosfeld. Described as an *I Love Lucy* coat!

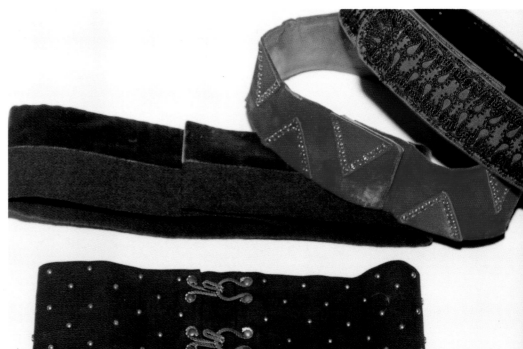

Ca. 1965 assortment of "designer" belts, including an elastic "cinch" belt, a cashmere and silk velvet wide belt, a satin and velvet wide belt, trimmed with red "stones," and a red satin belt, embroidered in black.

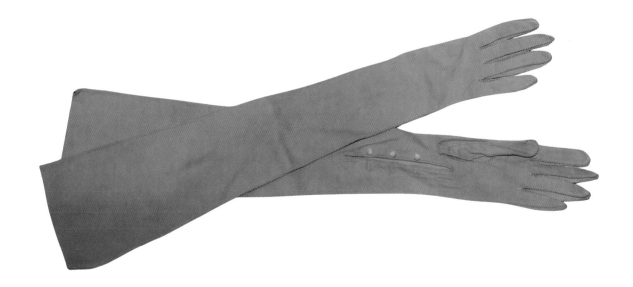

Ca. 1945 over-the-elbow blue kidskin gloves. Fashion gloves are virtually obsolete; only functional gloves for weather protection and sports remain.

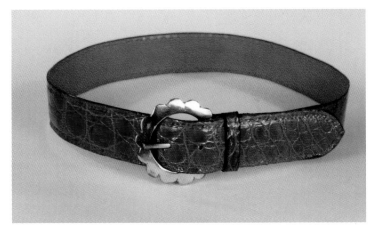

Ca. 1955 red alligator belt, with a brass buckle.

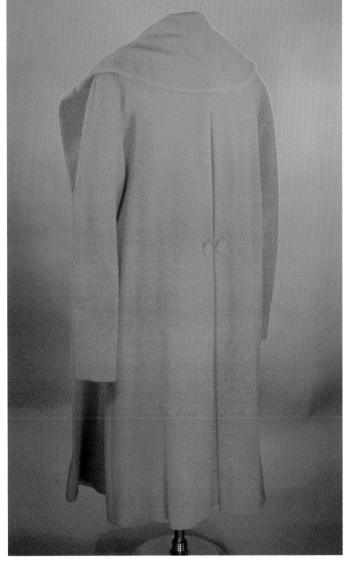

Ca. 1950 rose wool and cashmere wrap coat, photographed to show the pleated back with two covered buttons; satin lined.

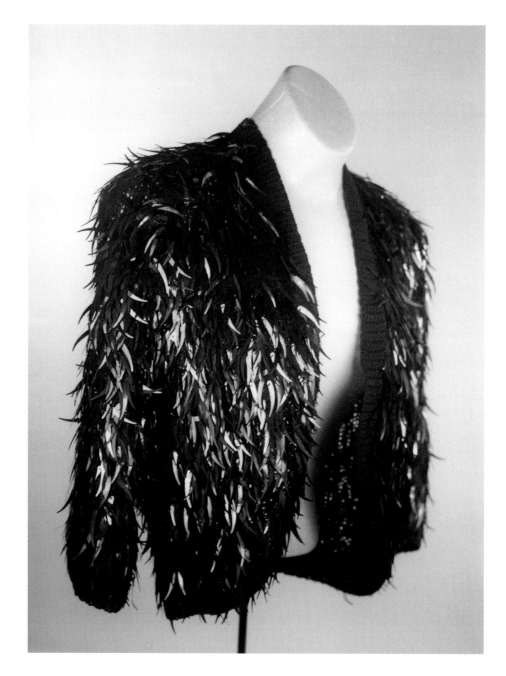

Ca. 1955 black sweater jacket, decorated all over with
elongated black sequins.

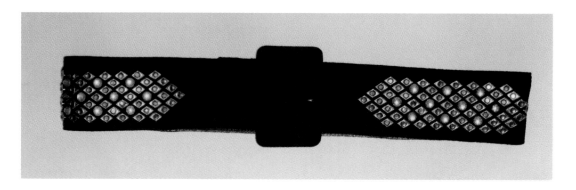

Ca. 1940 black crepe belt, decorated with blue glass "stones"
and brass diamonds.

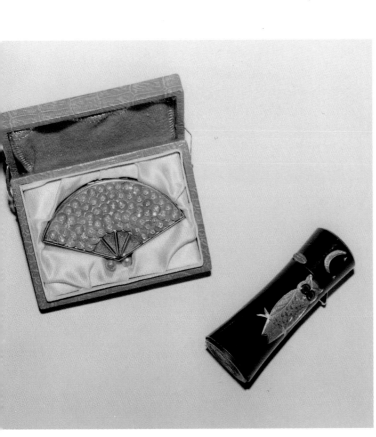

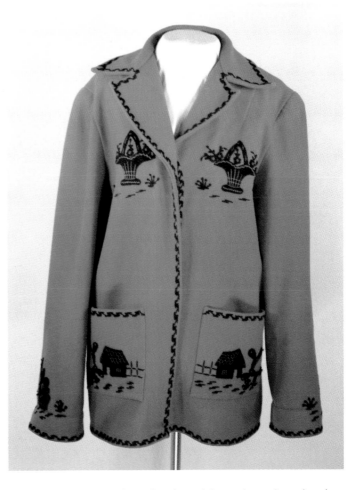

Ca. 1960 purse accessories; a compact shaped like a fan, decorated with blue sequins; a black Lucite lighter with metal inlay in the shape of an owl, below a crescent-shaped "moon." Purse accessories have been popular since the 1920s, but have become less elaborate and more functional in recent years.

Ca. 1950 aqua wool flannel jacket, elaborately appliquéd with black felt designs, front and back; collar and lapels embroidered with black wool thread; unlined; labeled Creaciones Berti, Monterrey. Jackets of this type were imported from Mexico in the early 1950s; most embroidered with more than one color. This is a particularly nice example of the type.

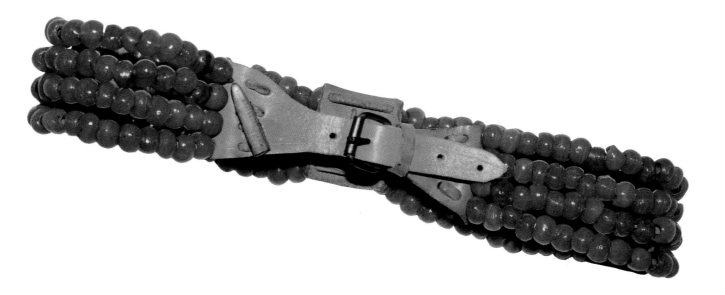

Ca. 1965 belt made up of four rows of blue ceramic beads, with a tan leather strap and brass buckle.

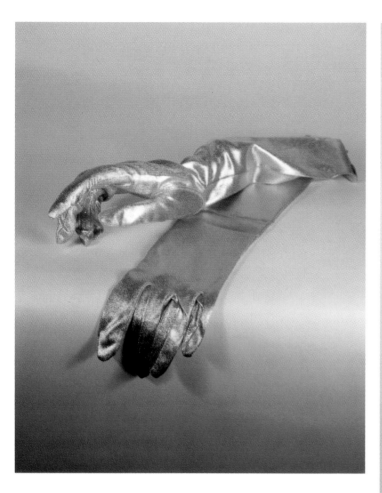

Ca. 1955 gold lamé long gloves.

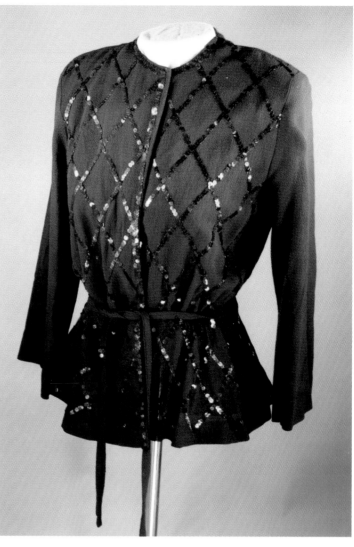

Ca. 1940 black crepe jacket, decorated with diagonally crossing rows of sequins; gathered and belted at the waist; large shoulder pads.

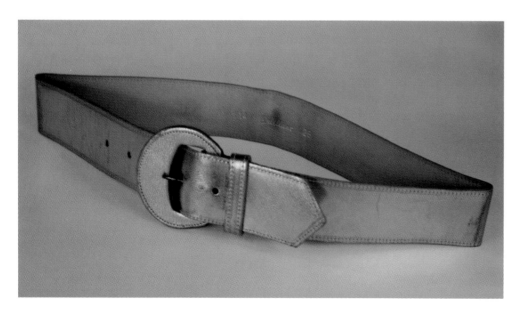

Ca. 1930 gold leather belt.

1930s rayon/silk printed crepe

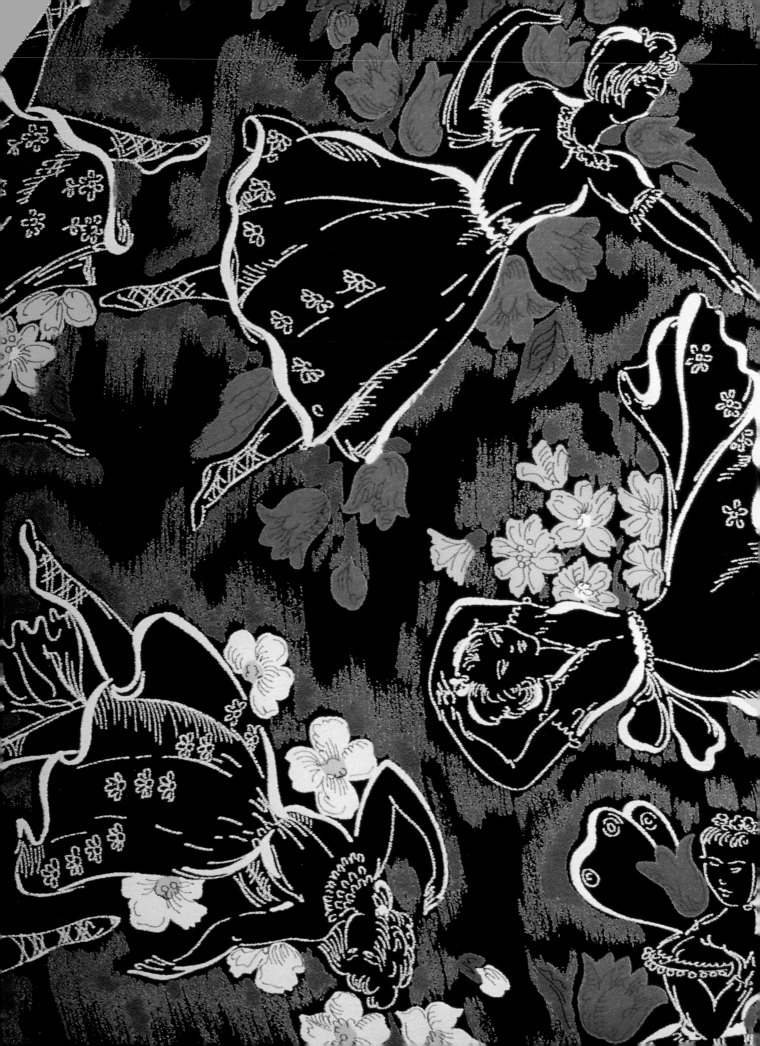

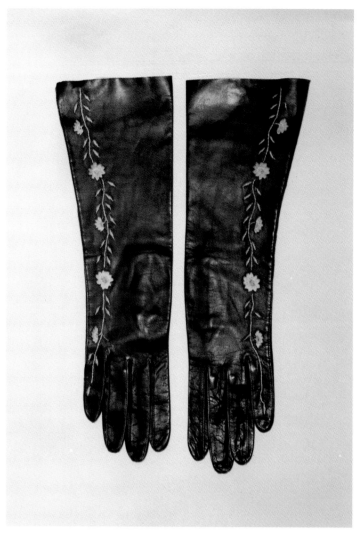

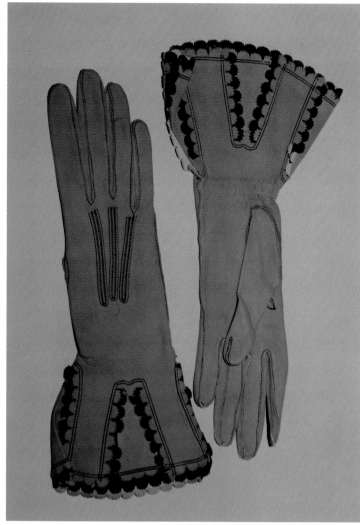

Ca. 1950 black kidskin gloves, embroidered with flowers.

Ca. 1920 tan suede riding gloves, with elaborate brown suede detailing, showing a "pinking" edge; Made in France.

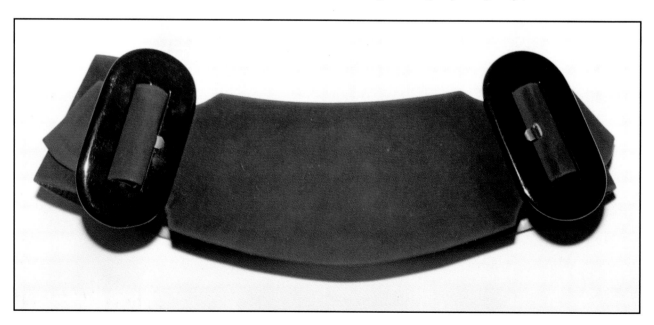

Ca. 1965 wide black kidskin belt, with two large, plastic buckles; stamped Made In Austria.

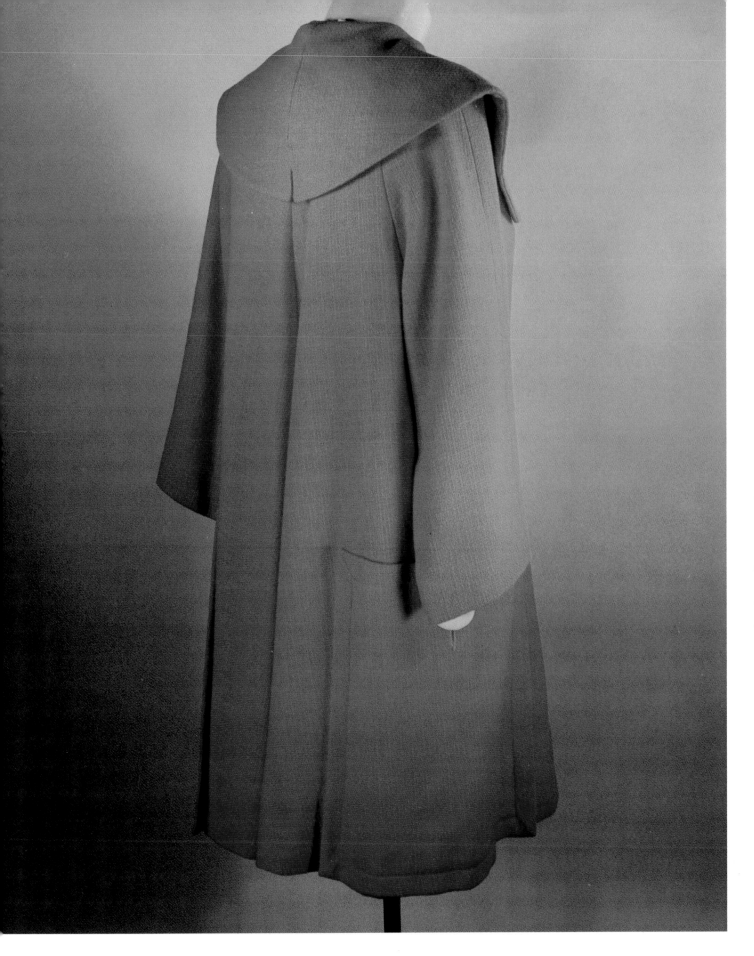

Ca. 1955 pink wool swing coat, with an ample collar, over-
sized pockets, and large, white plastic buttons; taffeta lined.

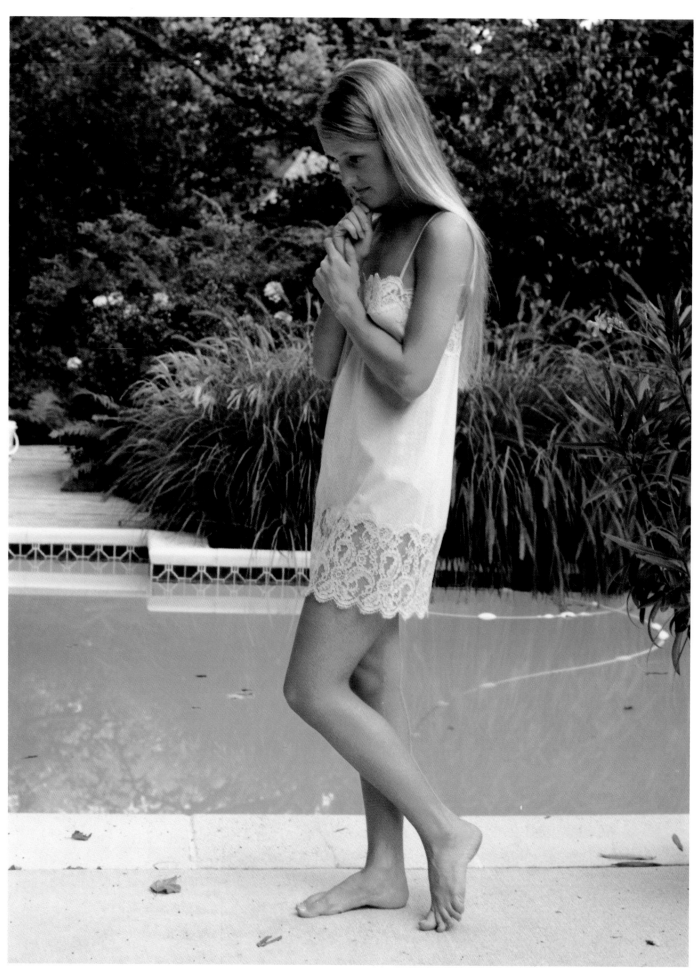

Chapter 3

The Fashion Industry

Couture is still alive and well, and the fashion industry is one of the most important industries in the world today. However, collecting and speculating in *vintage* couture is not for the unknowledgable or the faint of heart. Like any other field of art collecting, it is sensitive to trends in the market, the politics of what is being sold at the major auction houses and shown at the major museums, as well as the trends in *new* clothing for the season. It may even be affected by current films, celebrity deaths, and a host of factors as uncontrollable as the weather. A collector is wise who considers the intrinsic merit of the individual piece. An individual who collects *vintage* couture must know fashion history, fabric, and design, as well as the nature of the designer's contribution and the evolution of that designer's style and exact production. Then, after all this, have access to the clothes!

Occasionally, a vintage clothing buyer may run across a couture piece at a bargain price, but generally such labels as Callot Soeurs, Cristobal Balenciaga, Mariano Fortuny, Paul Poiret, Madeleine Vionnet, and Charles Frederick Worth can only be found through dealers who specialize in the highest level couture. It is more probable to see the work of these designers in the fashion collections of major museums. How wearable are these clothes? Although the designs of the great couturiers of the world were made to be worn, it would be unwise to wear such clothing at this time in history, considering how rare and extremely valuable it is. In the event that a couturier dies, and his or her fashion house is closed for good, that couturier's label becomes instantly more valuable. Although a few private collectors have significant collections of couture, much of it in good condition has been preserved in museum collections.

There is always a fine line between preservation and use. Some of us collect and use the very best examples of antique furniture, but with clothing and textiles the standard is somewhat different. The object itself is far less durable. A gabardine jacket that is sixty years old, with an "off-the-rack" label, may be very wearable for a very long time with proper storage and cleaning. It can be recycled and appreciated for another generation of use. I have no problem with wearing couture level clothing designed in the 1950s and 1960s, if it is not fragile, but this is a matter of personal taste and point of view.

The fashion industry is an excellent example of the marriage of art and industry--and it is not always a happy union! As consumers of fashion, influenced by trends and advertising, we have precious little knowledge about the "inner workings" of the industry. Vintage clothing and accessories are of considerable interest to many contemporary designers. The following conversation with Louise Stewart relates some interesting "insider" information about the fashion industry. Louise is a graduate of Drexel University's Fashion Design Program and is currently working as a design coordinator for a company that specializes in "ready-to-wear" fashions.

Why did you decide to major in fashion design?

I'd been sewing since fourth grade. My middle name was for an aunt, Mary, who was a seamstress in Philadelphia, and I wore many garments she made.

How important are the skills learned in design programs at the college level?

Ca. 1960 lace-edged, white, silk mini-slip. *Modeled by Marcie Behanna.*

Very important in terms of technical skills, and equally important in teaching an "eye" for design.

What makes a great design?

Such things as fabric choice, fit, image.

Who is your favorite designer of all time?

Cristobal Balenciaga...I just feel he could do it all.

Who is your favorite contemporary designer?

Calvin Klein. He has a number of lines, including Calvin Klein Sport, and has great marketing. He's been on the top for a very long time!

What inspires designers? How common is it to use vintage pieces for inspiration?

Inspiration is very individual. Some designers have extensive libraries; others have people out looking for ideas and trends, and vintage clothing is part of it. Designers often use vintage couture to "down-line." (less expensive copy)

How does one become a well-known designer?

There are many elements involved over which you have no control. Organizational skills are important...and being at the right place at the right time. The individual designer is less important now than in the past. Buyers are taking a major role. They may say, "put a body in this dress (last year's style), but change the print."

Without getting too technical, what are the steps in the production of a garment?

Idea, sketch, pattern is made, garment is made (in the goods chosen for production, not in muslin), fitting, second fitting, corrections are made, and garment is put into production.

How important are the spring/fall fashion shows in Paris?

Very important for trend-setting and name-getting. These shows add a lot of excitement to the field!

Is the production schedule also based on the seasons of the year?

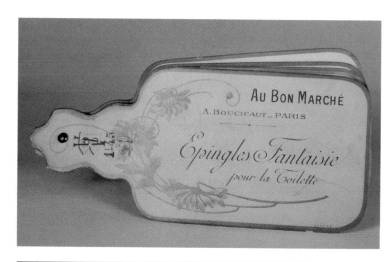

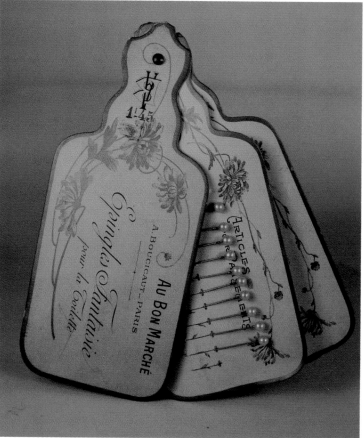

A paper fan of ca. 1890 lingerie pins of all types, each identified; stamped Au Bon Marche, A. Boucicaut-Paris; Epingles Fantaisie pour la Toilette.

In terms of production it's on-going, but they still do four major lines each year and four major market weeks--fall, holiday, trans, and summer.

I'm assuming that "holiday" relates to party dresses and gowns, but what is "trans?"

"Trans" means transitional. It used to have to do with resort and cruise wear. I'm not sure who's going on cruises!

What causes a trend in fashion?

Young people start the trends, bucking the establishment. The market spots the new trend and jumps on it! Rumors are that some designers have people spotting and following around the "cool" kids, so that they can jump on these trends.

Is the market for women's clothing larger than for men's?

Definitely...women follow the trends. Men's clothing has made great leaps in recent years, especially in sports' clothing, but still men wear the same suits.

How important is the computer in the field today?

Tremendously important in terms of every aspect of manufacturing, inventory, and ticketing.

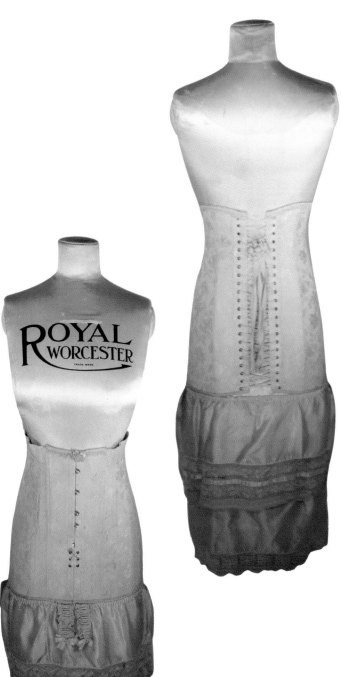

Ca. 1890 silk corset form and corset; stamped Royal Worcester Trade Mark; below the corset are lace-trimmed, silk petticoats over a turned wooden base. Made as an advertising piece for the Royal Worcester Company, near Lehighton, Pennsylvania, in 1890, it remained at their offices until the company closed, apparently in the 1950s. *Purchased by Marlene Minnick from the company; author's collection.*

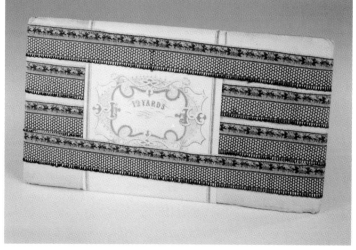

Twelve yards of ca. 1890 black silk lace ribbon, embroidered with roses.

127

Are there many couturiers in contemporary society?

No. Although it takes a great many people to make even one shirt today, great sewing is a lost art. Very few have the skills to do it. Not as much time is put into the individual piece as it was in the past.

Who is actually making the clothes now? How much is made overseas?

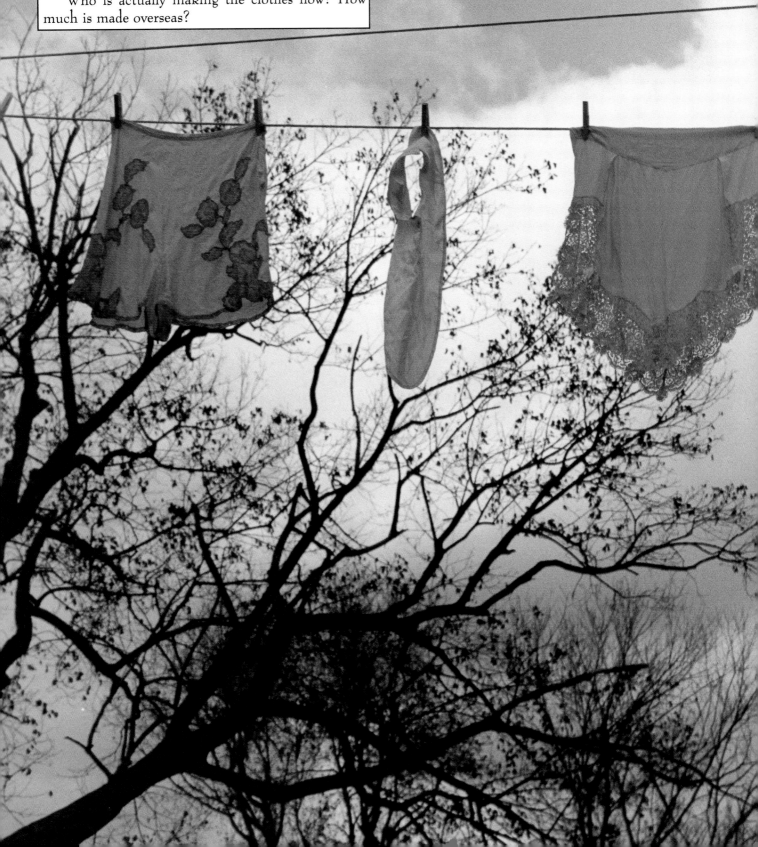

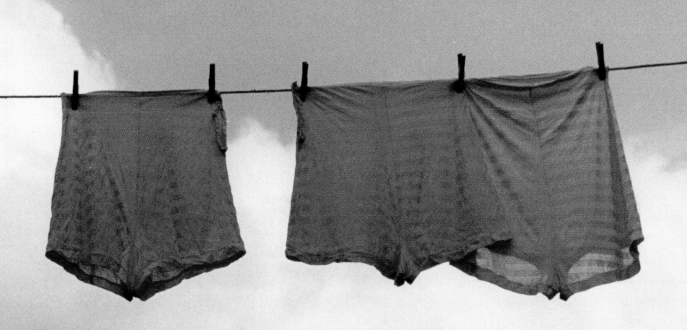

Ca. 1930 silk panties; some with lace edging or applique.

The majority of clothes are being made overseas. "Last resorts" (needed it yesterday and no one else would take the job) and "quick turn-arounds," (has to be done immediately) are usually manufactured in the states.

Is sportswear typically American?

Americans like to dress informally, yes, but at this point, wearing sportswear is global!

Louise Stewart's remarks about sewing as a "lost art," and the inability and unwillingness of contemporary manufacturers to put significant time into the individual piece, strengthens the supposition of collectors of vintage "ready-to-wear" and couture clothing that the old is significantly different from the new. Many "off-the-rack" vintage pieces are beautifully sewn and elaborately detailed, when compared with similar items manufactured today.

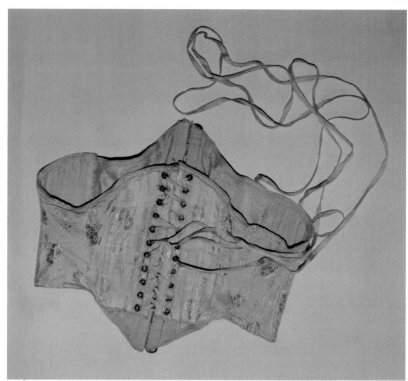

Ca. 1947 cotton brocade waist corset; labeled Waspies, By Roth Creations. There was an attempt to popularize the "wasp waist" (named for the insect with a tiny waist) which had been fashionable during the 1890s.

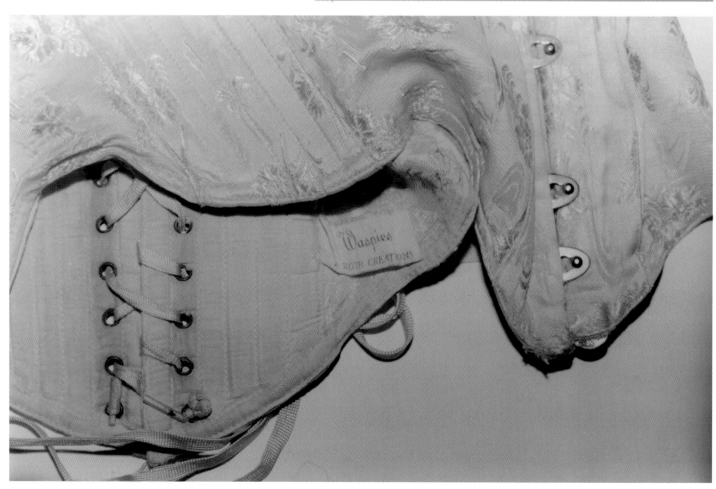

Ca. 1930 flannel robe in shades of tan and blue, with a blue silk braided sash and blue silk piping on the lapels, cuffs, and pockets. *Modeled by Kim Hemingway.*

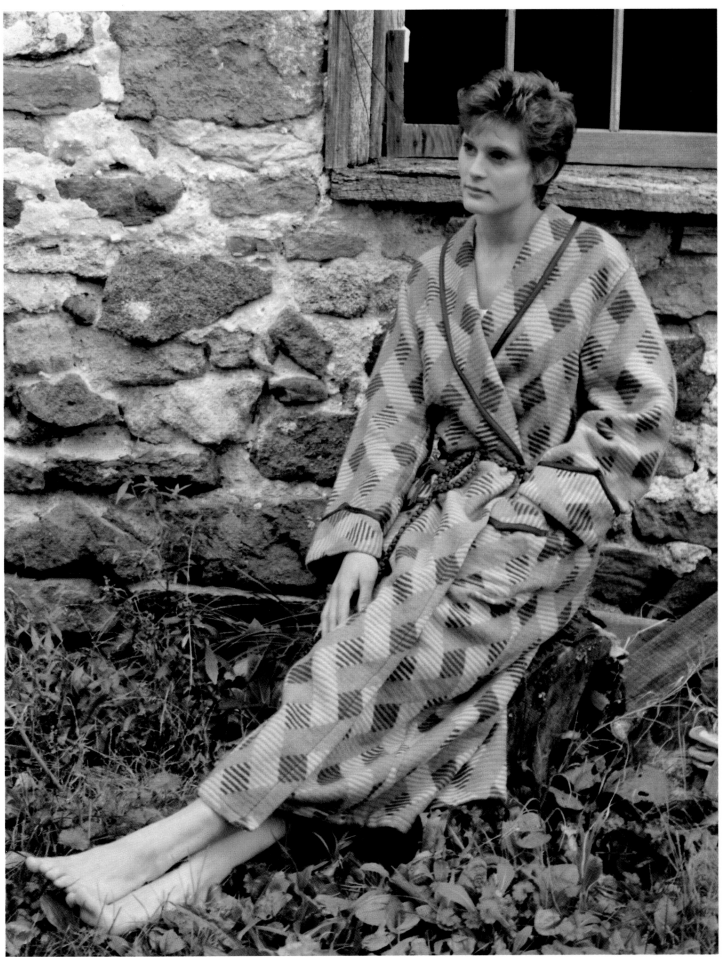

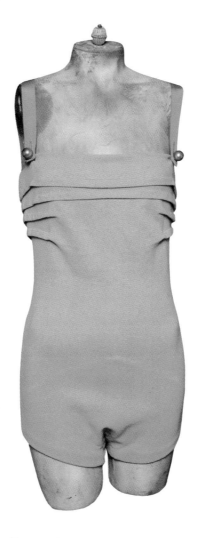

Ca. 1920 red silk, Spanish shawl embroidered in shades of blue, gold, and mauve. *Modeled by Marcie Behanna.*

Ca. 1940 yellow, wool jersey swimsuit with two horizontal pleats across the top and two, large, round brass buttons attaching the straps; labeled Claire McCardell. *Courtesy of Mark Walsh. Photograph by Kelly Wright.*

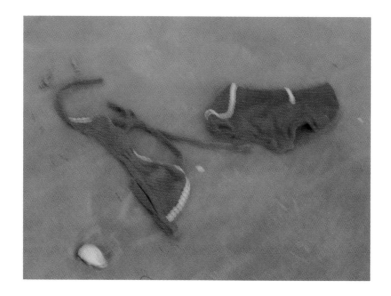

Ca. 1950 red, cotton terry cloth, two-piece swimsuit trimmed with white braid and lined with white cotton jersey.

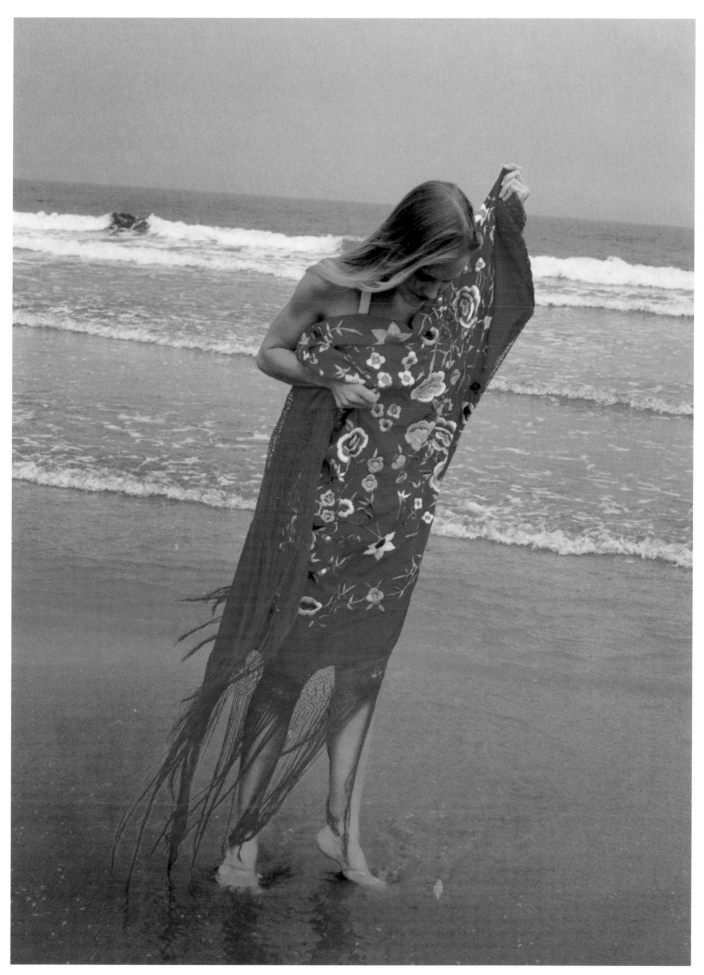

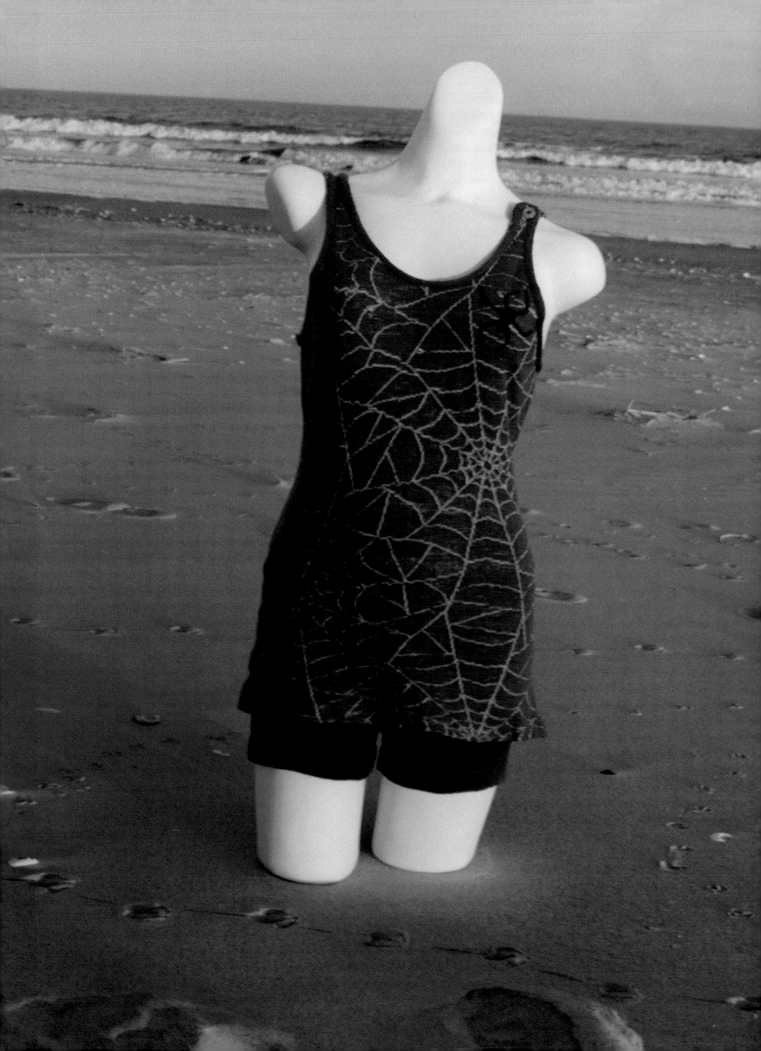

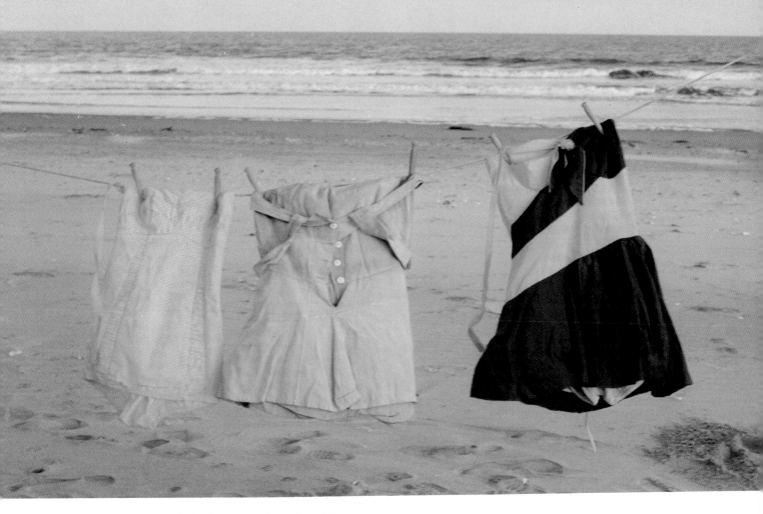

Ca. 1950 swimsuits on a clothesline, including, from left to right, a yellow acetate swimsuit labeled sea nymph, glamour suit by jordan, Made of Acetate Cotton Rubber; a pale green rayon faille, skirted swimsuit; a green and yellow spandex skirted swimsuit, labeled Jantzen.

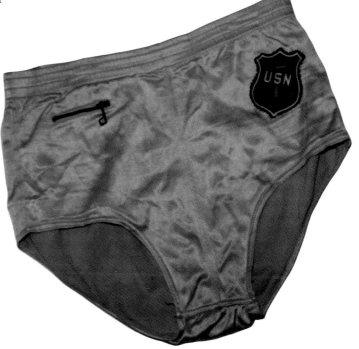

Ca. 1920 blue, wool swimsuit with a "spiders on a web" design: three black spiders on chartreuse spider webs, two on the front and one on the back; labeled U. S. A., slip into a Bradley, and out of doors. An early "spider woman" suit!

Ca. 1935 man's, ivory satin, swim trunks with "USN" patch; zippered front pocket.

135

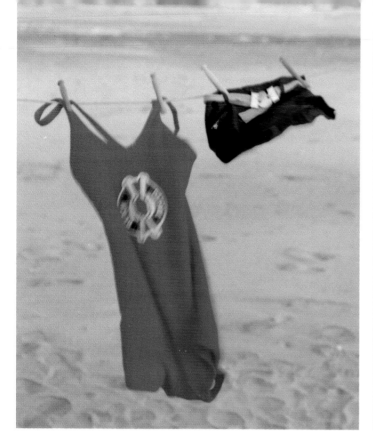

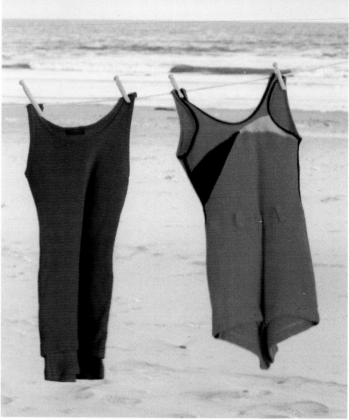

Ca. 1930 swimsuits on a clothesline, from left to right, red wool tank suit, with an emblem on front, displaying "crossed oars," and the letters M. C. B. P. Beach Patrol; and maroon wool swim trunks, with a zipper pocket, and a cotton belt which has an elaborate metal buckle, with a "diving figure" on it. Blowing in the wind!

Ca. 1928 maroon wool swimsuit, labeled AMHO, American Hosiery Co., and red wool swimsuit trimmed with pale green and navy blue.

Ca. 1925 black and rose, cotton knit stockings with white horizontal stripes.

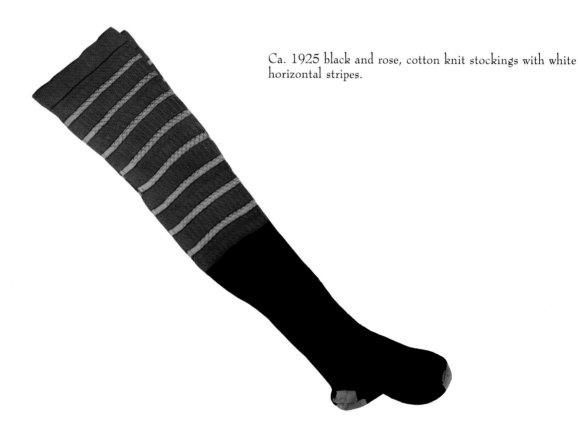

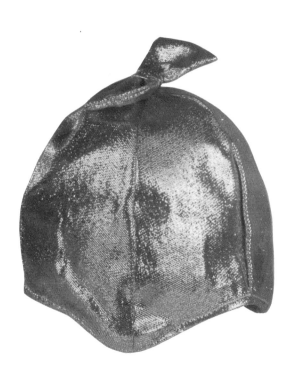

Ca. 1958 silver metallic, rubber bathing cap. *Courtesy of Janet Milburn.*

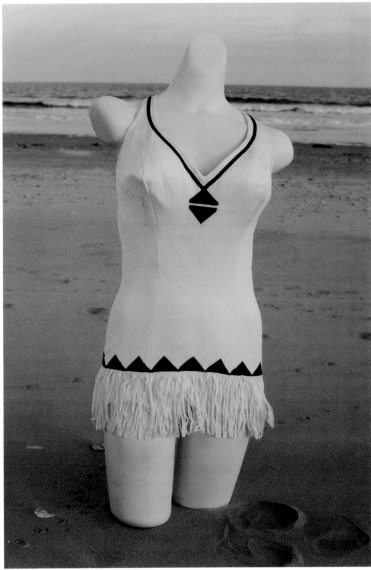

Ca. 1955 white Spandex swimsuit trimmed with navy blue braid and navy blue Latex triangles and rayon fringe; labeled DeWeese Design.

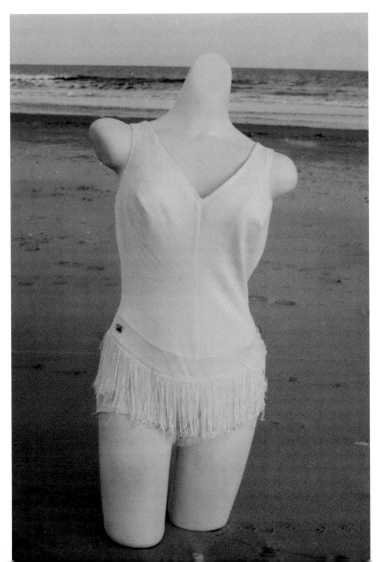

Ca. 1955 white Spandex swimsuit trimmed with rayon fringe; two pyramid-shaped brass buttons decorate the hipline.

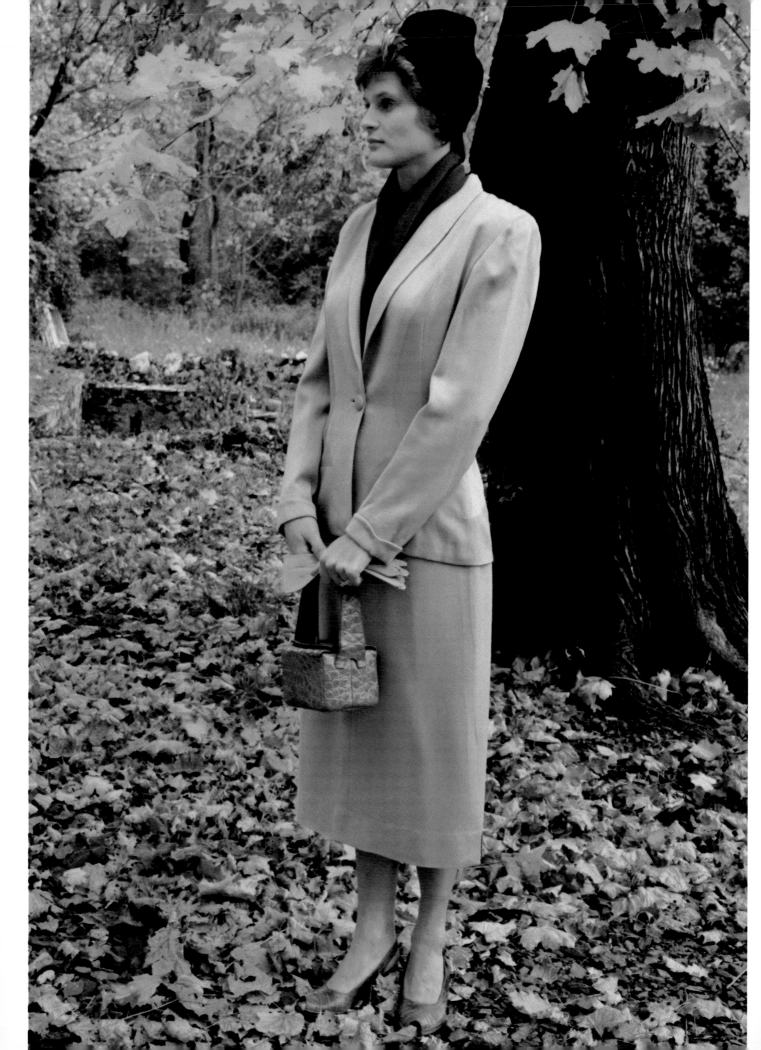

Chapter 4
Handbags

The handbag is an accessory which makes it possible to carry a number of items, essential for women in recent years, such as keys, check books, credit cards, and all kinds of unmentionables. The handbag, pocketbook, purse, or "bag" which women carry today is larger than it has ever been in history. Some women carry giant back packs or shoulder bags, which function as lifestyle utility bags. Handbags of the past were far more diminutive!

Throughout the centuries men have had folding pocketbooks or wallets to carry their valuable papers and money. The aulmoniere, a small leather pouch, was worn suspended from a man's girdle during the 13th to the 16th centuries. Women used pockets, separate from their clothing, attached to their waists by drawstrings, to carry items useful in performing their household chores during the late 18th and into the 19th centuries. The reticule, a small, elongated bag was carried by women, from the late 19th to the early 20th century. During the late 19th century, various types of handbags were carried, especially for traveling. By the 1920s, handbags were a necessity.

Vintage Style focuses on handbags, from 1930 to 1960, that are available to the collector and at the same time special in terms of material and design. Handbags included in the book are useable, or "wearable," styles.

Vintage handbags come in many materials, including leather, plastic, fabric, vinyl, metal, canvas, straw, and patent leather. The box handbag, which became popular in the late 1940s and continued to be popular throughout the 1950s, was made in every imaginable material. Since the box style has a rigid frame, similar to a small suitcase or lunch box, it is possible to cover the frame with materials of all kinds. Particularly fashionable during the 1950s were box style handbags covered with the skins of reptiles-- lizard, crocodile, snake, and alligator. The bracelet handbag, also popular in the 1950s, is a soft pouch bag made of leather or fabric, with or without a frame, with one or two bangle bracelets as handles.

Ca. 1940 beige, wool, gabardine suit; jacket in two tones of beige gabardine, one a shade darker than the other; lined with beige crepe; labeled Victor Alexander, a California Creator, Goodman's, Lincoln Road; worn with box style, tan alligator pocketbook, matching alligator pumps, and a brown, felt, period hat. *Modeled by Kim Hemingway.*

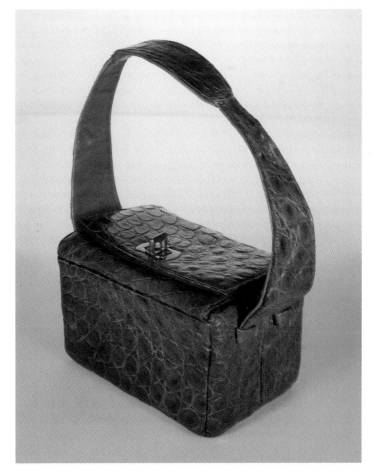

Ca. 1950 light brown, alligator, box-style pocketbook; overflap with small, brass turnstile clasp and leather lining; strap lined in brown faille. A very nice example of a box style!

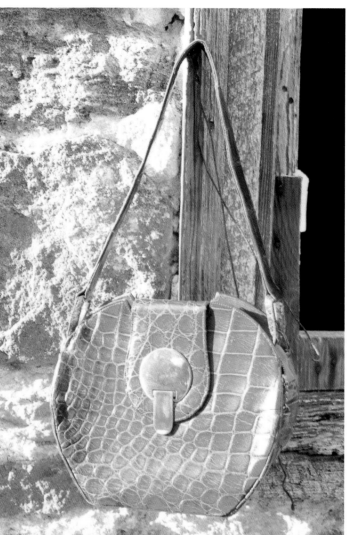

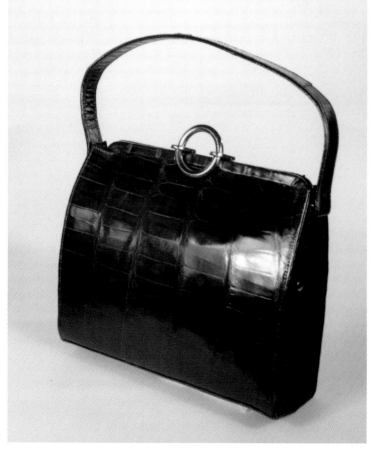

Ca. 1955 large, dark brown, alligator pocketbook lined with light beige kidskin. A beautiful example of its type.

Ca. 1940 brown, alligator pocketbook with unusual brass clasp and shoulder strap; leather lined; stamped Deitsch in gold. A great style!

Ca. 1955 brown crocodile pocketbook lined with light beige kidskin; elaborate brass clasp. A beautifully made and high quality pocketbook.

The clutch handbag is perhaps the most popular vintage style. Rectangular, without a handle, the clutch may be made in various materials and with all kinds of decoration, including all over beading. Some clutch pocketbooks have back-straps to make carrying easier. The fold-over clutch is a variation, designed to be folded over double and carried under the arm.

The mesh handbag is made up of tiny links of metal joined to make a flexible bag. Popular in the early 1900s, sometimes with a sterling silver top and chain, or with an enameled design on the links, the mesh handbag became larger in the 1940s, with large white, enameled links and a white plastic frame. The interchangeable handbag appeared during the 1950s. A complete handbag with extra covers that snap or button on to change fabric or color, the style became particularly popular with travelers. The minaudiere is a small, rigid metal evening bag used to hold cosmetics. Derived from the French word "simper," which means "smirk," this style was popularized by Cartier in New York. Many of these small oval, oblong, or square handbags are engraved with floral designs or set with jewels. Styles that are self-explanatory include the shoulder bag, the pouch, the barrel, the tote, and the accordion.

Accessories' designers often look to the past for inspiration. Collectors and fashionable women everywhere, shrewd enough to appreciate the beautiful craftsmanship of vintage handbags, ferret out these treasures at antiques markets, auctions, vintage clothing stores, and shows.

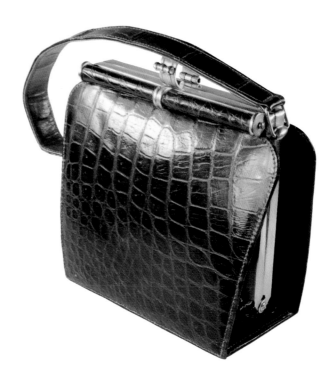

Ca. 1950 brown alligator pocketbook with an elaborate brass frame and clasp and lined in tan leather which is stamped in gold, Genuine Alligator, Hecho En Mexico; labeled Redrayes. Pocketbooks like this one were fashionable in the 1950s. A children's rhyme of the period says it all, "Here comes the doctor, here comes the nurse, here comes the lady with the alligator purse."

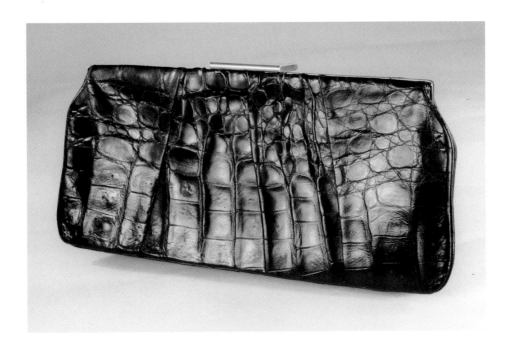

Ca. 1940 dark green crocodile, clutch style, pocketbook with a brass frame and clasp; lined with black faille.

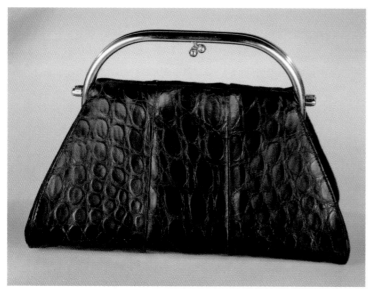

Ca. 1940 dark brown alligator pocketbook; brass rods slip through "pockets" and attach to the hoop-like handles to create the design, unusual catch at the top of the two brass handles; lined with brown faille.

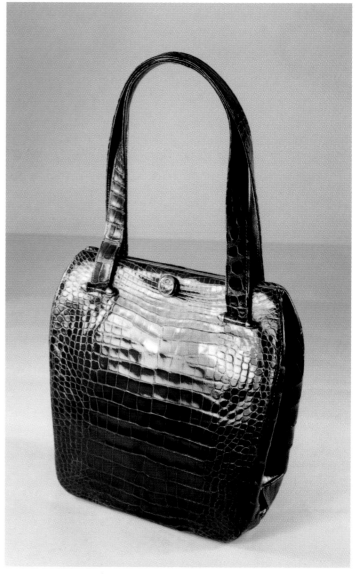

Ca. 1950 brown alligator pocketbook with a brass frame and a small, alligator "button" clasp; lined in brown leather and stamped Deitsch.

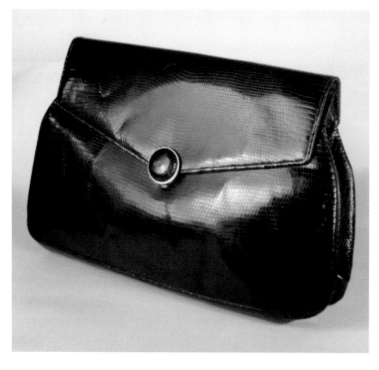

Ca. 1940 dark brown lizard, clutch pocketbook with back strap and a lift-up button closure, also covered in lizard; lined with tan suede and stamped Made in England, in gold.

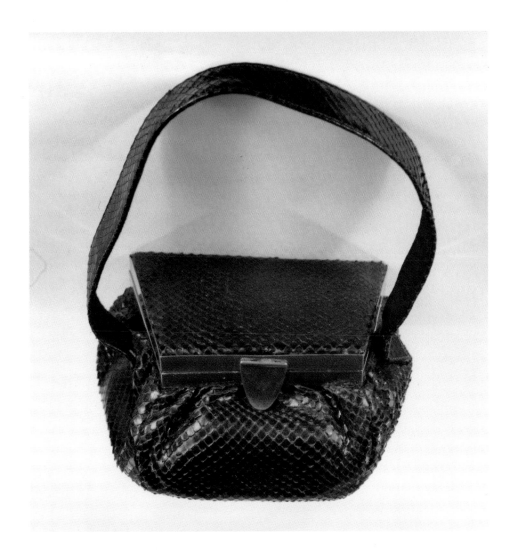

Ca. 1950 green snakeskin, pouch-style pocketbook on a brass
frame and lined with black faille; snakeskin handle.

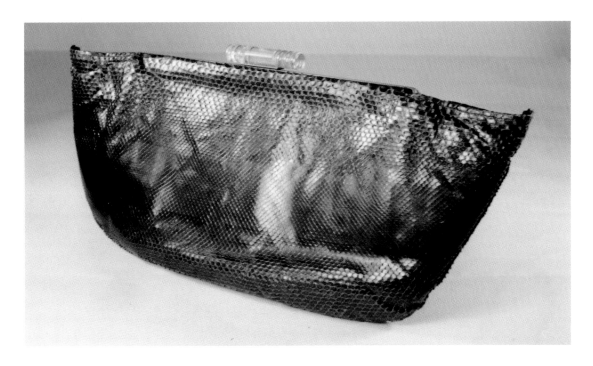

Ca.1940 green snakeskin, clutch-style pocketbook; brass
frame with a Bakelite clasp; lined with black silk taffeta.

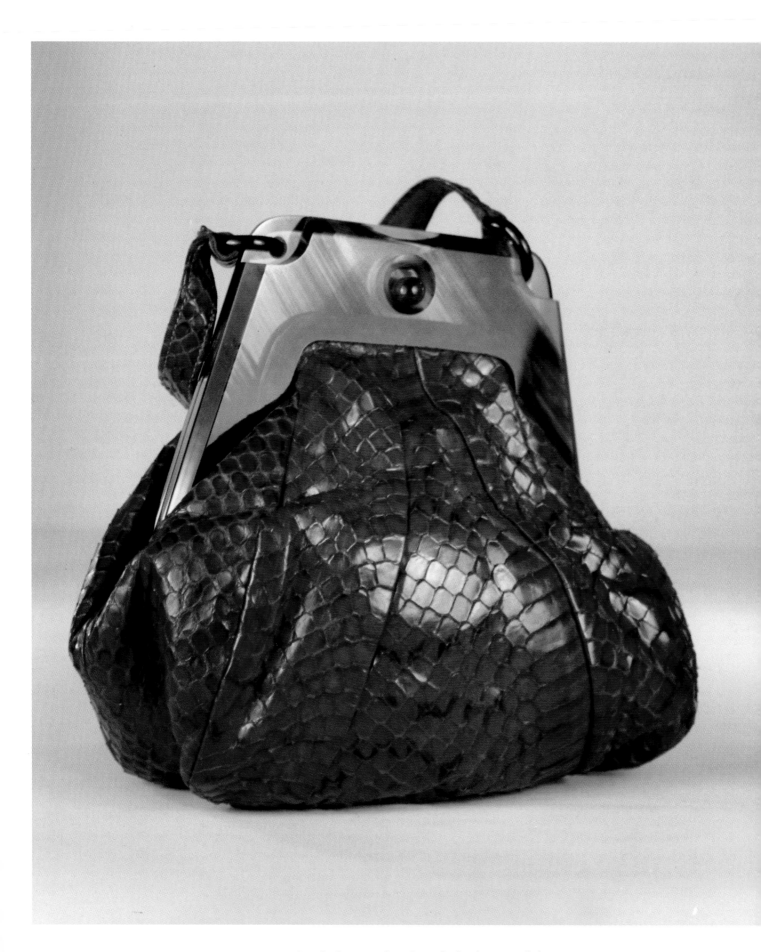

Ca. 1935 red snakeskin, pouch-style pocketbook on a Bakelite
frame; snakeskin handle; lined with black faille. Spectacular!

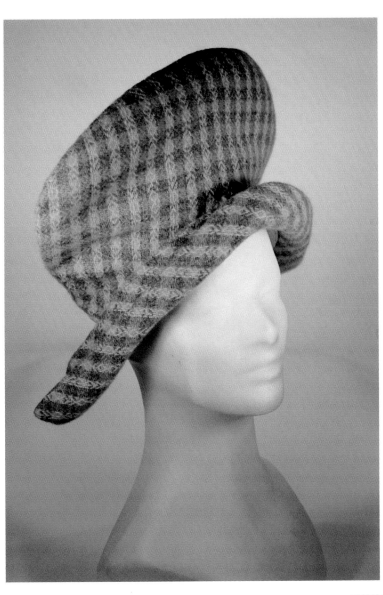

Ca. 1940 large, clutch-style pocketbook in gray and yellow wool tweed with a spring clasp and the letter "M" stitched on one side, lined with brown faille; shown with a matching hat labeled Millinery by Helen, 6005 Ogontz Ave., Phila.

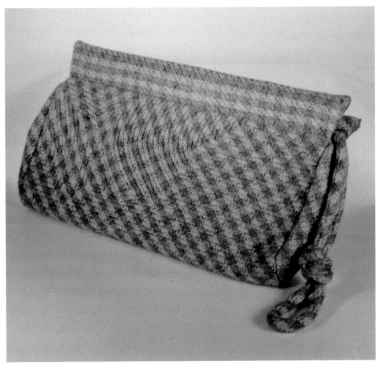

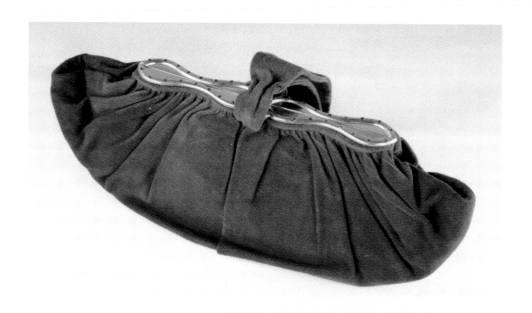

Ca. 1940 brown suede pocketbook gathered onto a brass frame and decorated with small, red, glass beads; single brown suede strap; stamped Koret.

Small booklet found inside the ca. 1940 brown suede, Koret pocketbook. The first page explains that Dick Koret designed various inside pockets of the handbag to hold your compact, lipstick, comb, "cigarette case or other out-sized impedimenta," as well as "the convenient little address book."

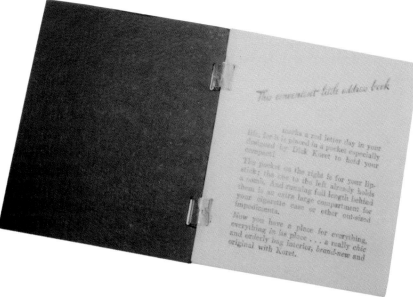

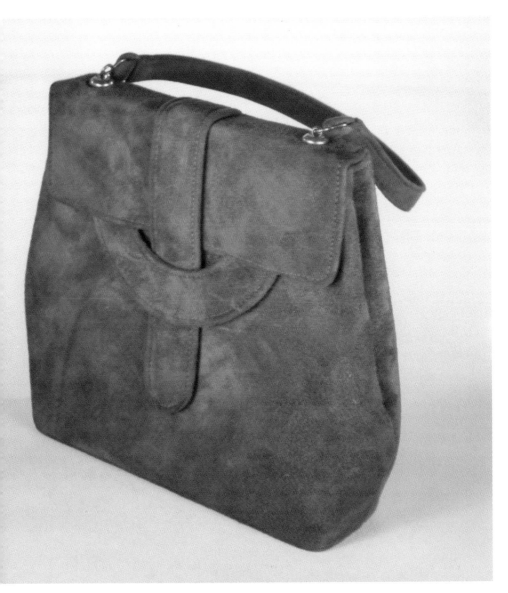

Ca. 1950 green suede pocketbook with a closure of the same material that passes through an attached loop.

Ca. 1940 brown flannel pocketbook designed with an unusual overlapping and gathering of material and a brass clasp; lined with brown faille and labeled Jenny, Paris, New York. *A gift from Donna Sigler.*

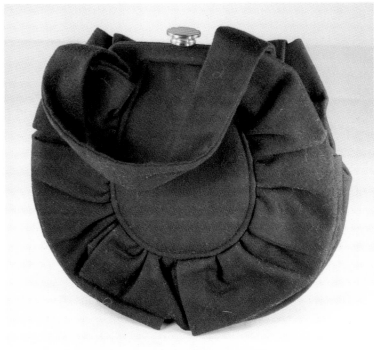

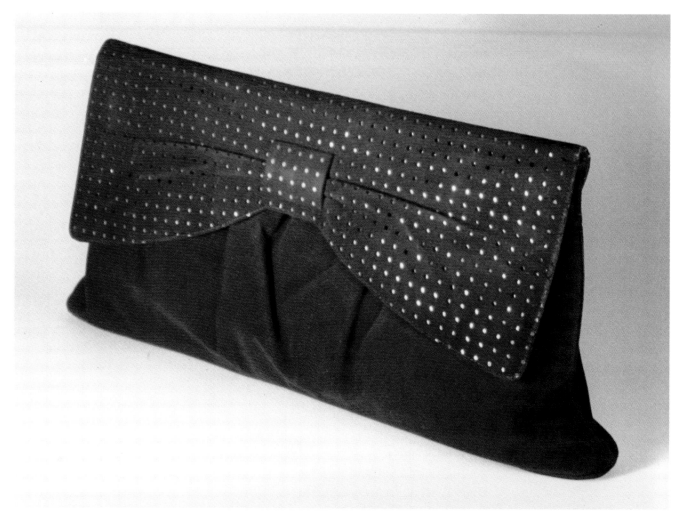

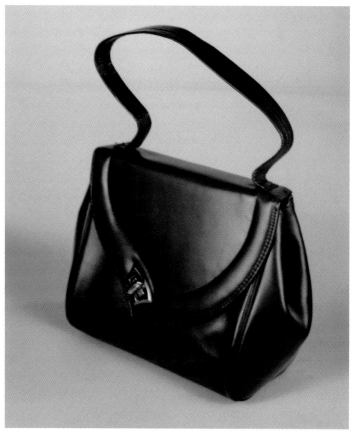

Ca. 1940 large, brown suede, clutch-style pocketbook. Underlying copper material shows through cut-out dots and the front is gathered into a bow design; lined with brown taffeta. *Courtesy of Roslyn Herman.*

Ca. 1940 green leather pocketbook; lined with black taffeta; labeled Marlow, Made in the U.S.A.

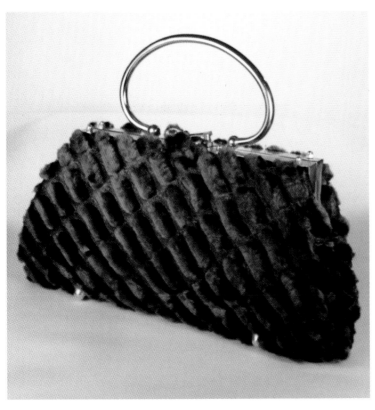

Ca. 1960 green chenille pocketbook; brass frame and modified bracelet-style handle, lined with black taffeta.

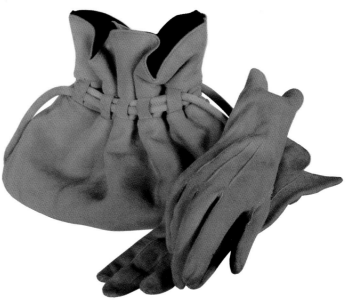

Ca. 1940 aqua suede, pouch-style pocketbook with matching suede gloves; drawstring closure; lined with black faille.

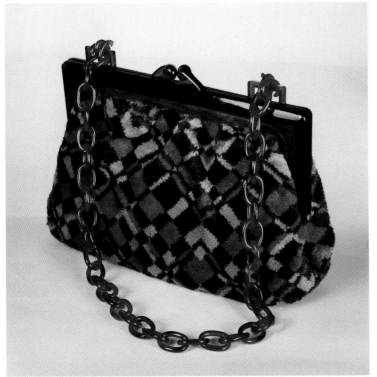

Ca. 1930 velvet, pouch-style pocketbook in shades of chestnut, dark brown, and yellow plaid; Bakelite frame and chain handle; lined with brown silk.

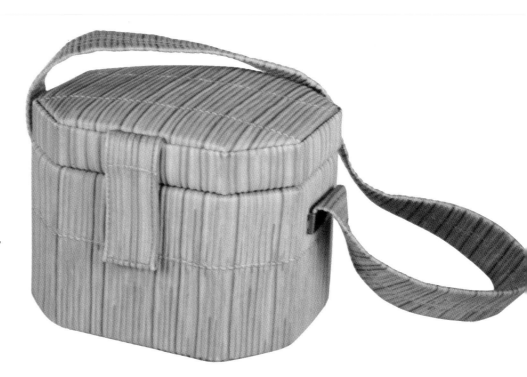

Ca. 1950 small, plastic, octagonal, box-style pocketbook designed to look like bundled reeds; mirror inside top and lined with black taffeta.

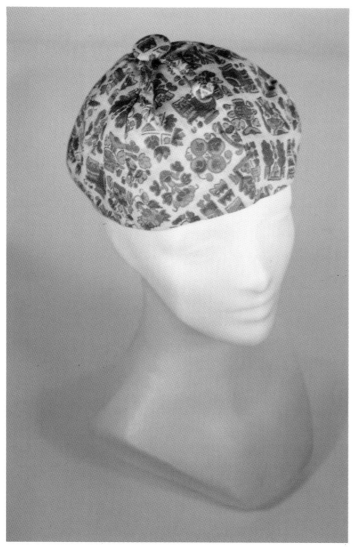

Ca. 1940 printed cotton, pouch-style pocketbook with a drawstring that passes through brass rings at the top; shown with a matching hat.

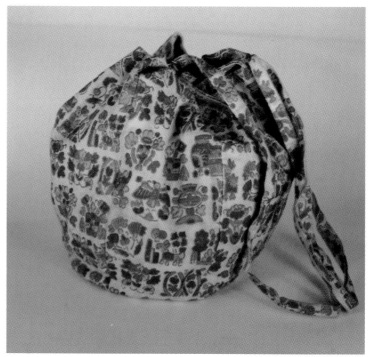

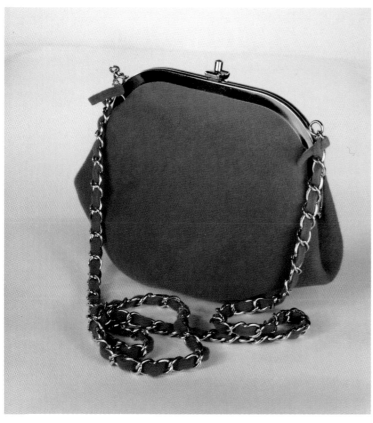

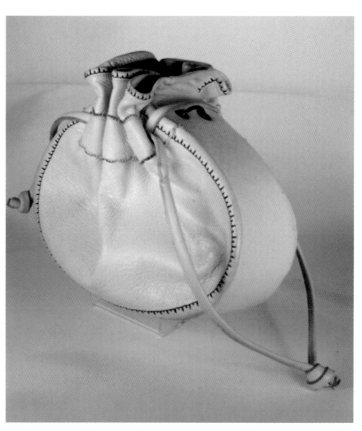

Ca. 1960 royal blue, velour, pouch-style pocketbook with a chain handle woven with the same material; lined with ivory satin.

Ca. 1940 beige leather pocketbook with rounded bottom and sides and drawstring closure; lined with black faille.

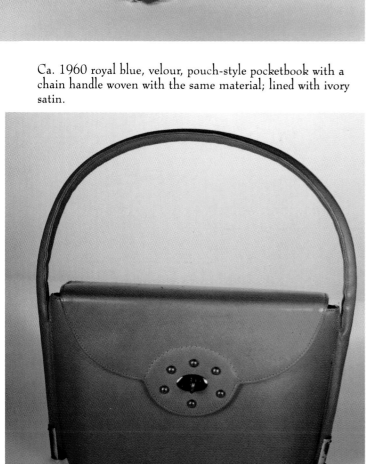

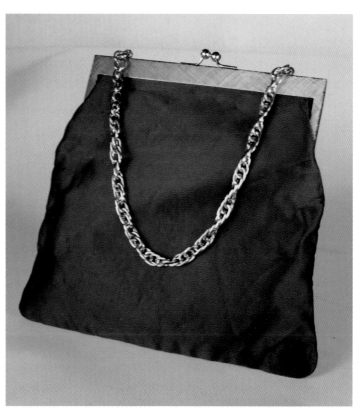

Ca. 1950 tan leather pocketbook; rigid, stand-up style with a hoop-like handle.

Ca. 1960 royal blue, silk, pouch-style pocketbook with brass frame and chain handle; lined with ivory silk; stamped Koret in gold.

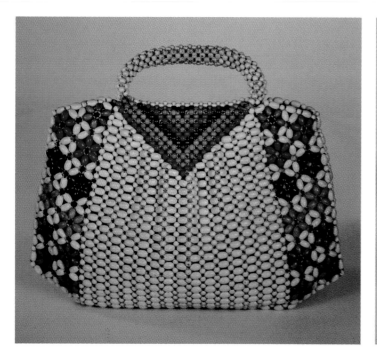

Ca. 1935 pocketbook made entirely of wooden beads in shades of red, green, gold, and white; beaded handle, zipper closure, and lined with silk taffeta.

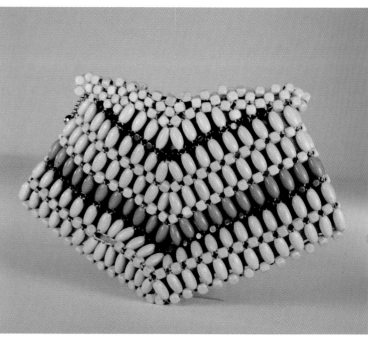

Ca. 1935 small, clutch-style pocketbook made entirely of wooden beads in pastel shades of green, yellow and pink, and contrasting strands of black and red beads; back strap, zipper closure, and lined with black faille.

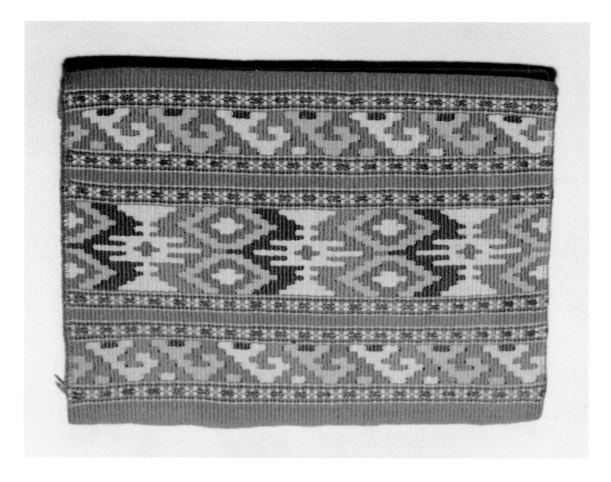

Ca. 1930 clutch-style pocketbook of woven cotton in shades of red, gold, blue and white; zipper closing; lined in ivory silk; zipper signed Ritsch.

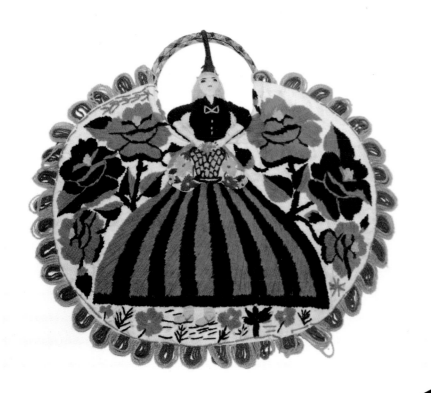

Ca. 1940 pouch-style pocketbook with bracelet handles decorated in crewel embroidery on a natural muslin base; shows the figure of a woman wearing a green and black skirt and holding flowers; additional green and black flowers are all around the figure; paper labeled Made in Madeira, Portugal.

Ca. 1930 printed linen, pouch-style pocketbook showing green parrots sitting on tree branches with pink and rose blooms against a mauve background, edged with black braid; handle of the same fabric and a black tassel. A great design!

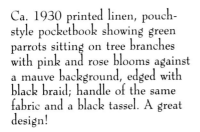

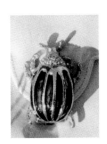

Ca. 1960 beige patent leather pocketbook with a brass and green enameled "beetle" clasp; lined with vinyl; long chain handle; stamped Robert Bestien Original.

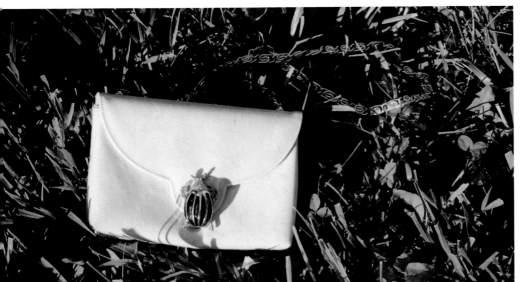

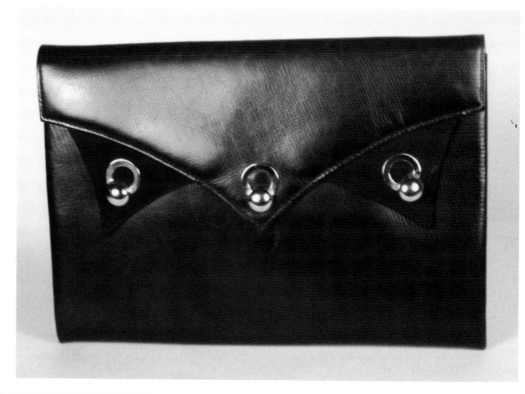

Ca. 1940 black leather clutch-style pocketbook with a back strap; decorated with three chrome rings and lined with black faille.

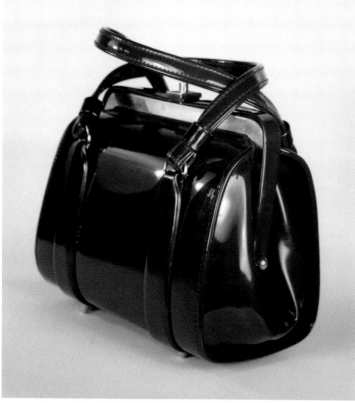

Ca. 1960 blue patent leather pocketbook with handles that extend around the case; chrome frame and clasp; labeled Empress.

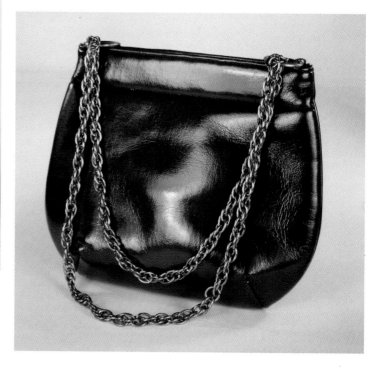

Ca, 1960 navy blue, soft vinyl, pouch-style pocketbook with a snap clasp and chain handle; lined with navy blue faille; labeled by Etra.

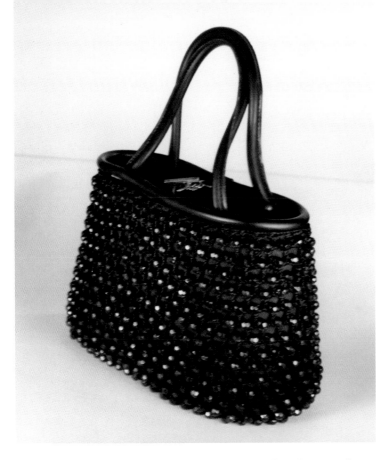

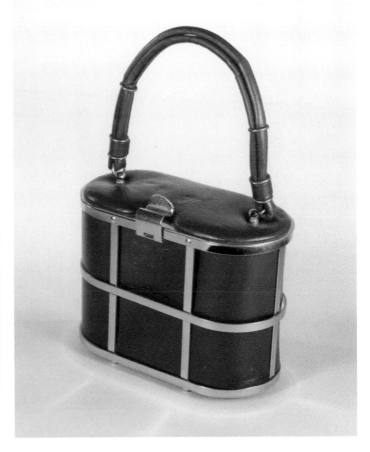

Ca. 1960 black leather, tote-style pocketbook with an overlay of black beaded net.

Ca. 1955 black patent leather, cylinder-style pocketbook constructed of vertical straps around an oval base; snap closure, lined with black faille.

Ca. 1955 oval cylinder-shaped, navy blue leather pocketbook with an outside brass cage and lined with navy blue faille.

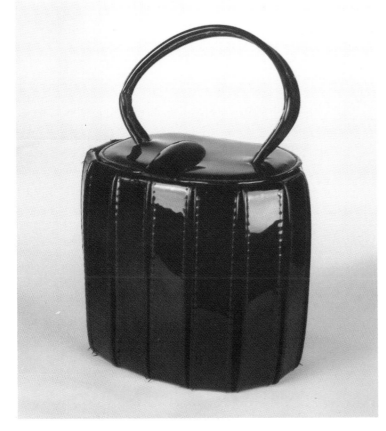

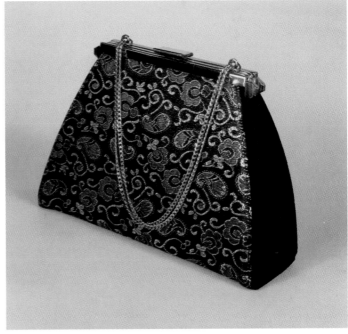

Ca. 1950 brocade over black faille interchangeable pocketbook; the outer cover comes off to expose another color; brass frame; chain handles.

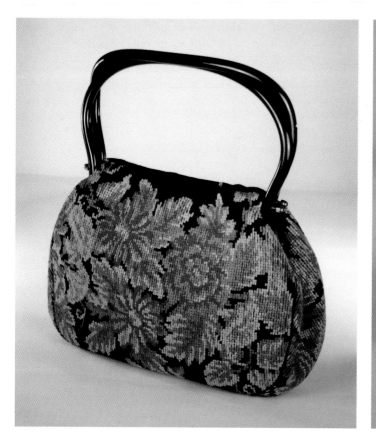

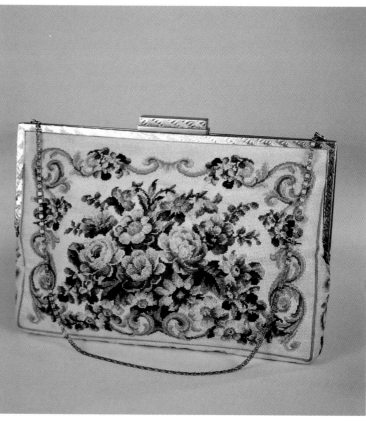

Ca. 1950 tapestry pocketbook in a floral design of rose, mauve, blue, and green on a black background; black plastic handles twist together; lined with black taffeta.

Ca. 1935 petit point tapestry pocketbook on brass, decorated frame; floral patterns in rose, blue, and gold on an ivory background; delicate chain handle; lined with silk satin.

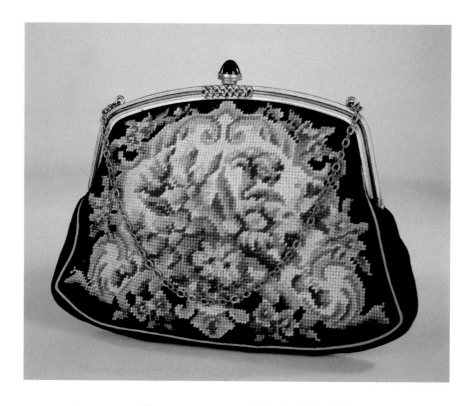

Ca. 1940 needlepoint tapestry pocketbook of floral design in shades of blue, rose, green, and white on a black background; enameled brass frame; clasp set with black onyx; lined with silk.

Ca. 1920 pale blue crocheted pocketbook with hundreds of horizontal rows of opalescent, oyster-white beads and a silver frame with elaborate filigree, and a chain handle; lined with pale blue silk.

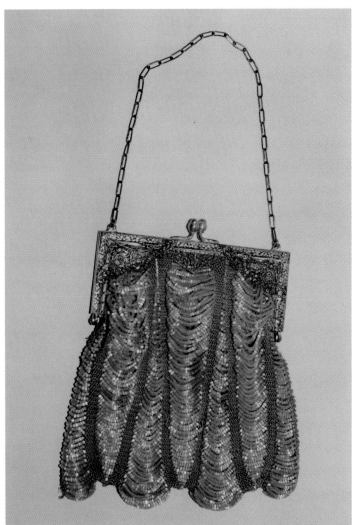

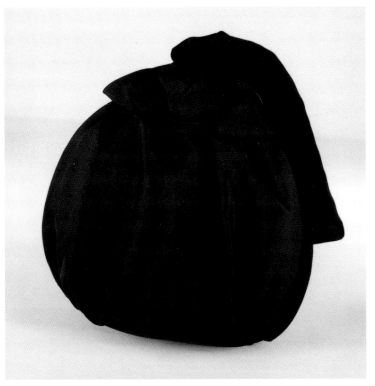

Ca. 1940 black silk evening pocketbook with a silk bracelet handle and top fabric folded to look like a rose. An amazing piece!

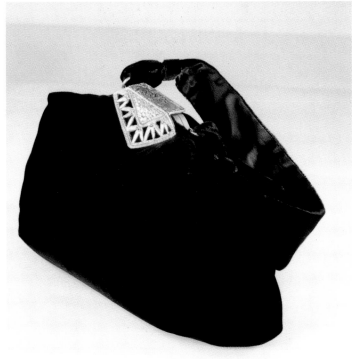

Ca. 1945 black silk velvet pocketbook with a brass frame and an unusual brass clasp; lined with black silk taffeta; velvet handle lined with black silk satin. A personal favorite because of its appealing texture and structure.

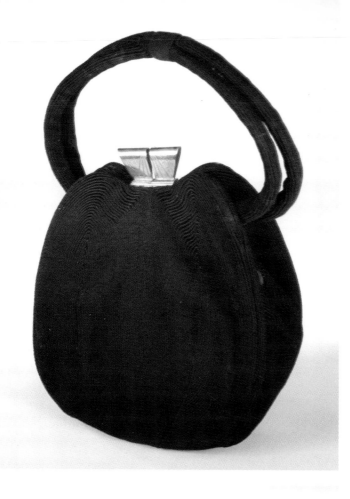

Ca. 1940 black cordé pocketbook with two cordé handles and a brass clasp with engraving; lined with black satin; stamped Genuine Paris Original.

Ca. 1940 elaborately layered, black cordé pocketbook with heavy brass frame and cordé handles that have a center crossing; lined with black satin.

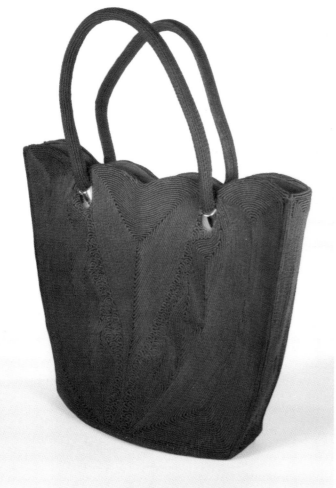

Ca. 1940 navy blue cordé pocketbook, tote style with brass handle attachments and zipper closing; labeled Genuine Cordé Creation.

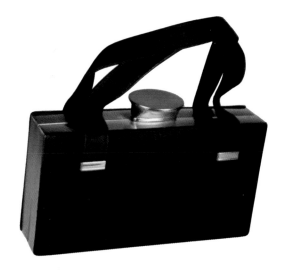

Ca. 1950 minaudiere covered with black silk; includes cosmetic cases for lipstick and powder and a cigarette case in brass. *Courtesy of Roslyn Herman.*

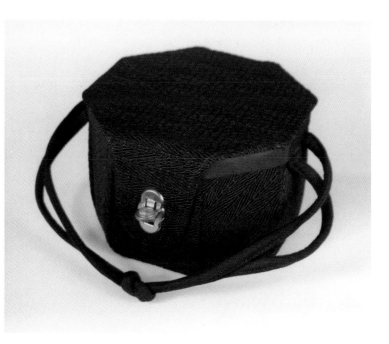

Ca. 1940 small, black cordé, octagonal box-style pocketbook with a knotted handle and a mirror inside the top.

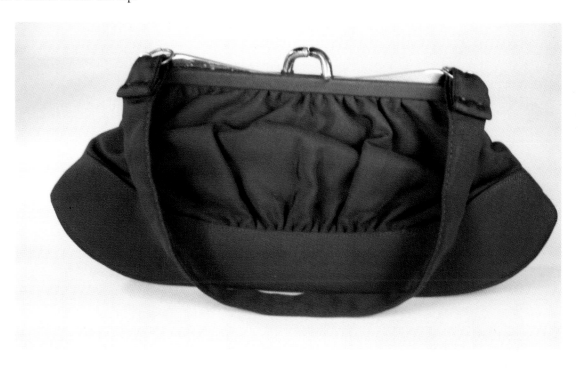

Ca. 1950 navy blue, silk faille pocketbook divided into two separate compartments, one lined in red silk and the other in navy silk; brass frame and clasp, labeled Koret.

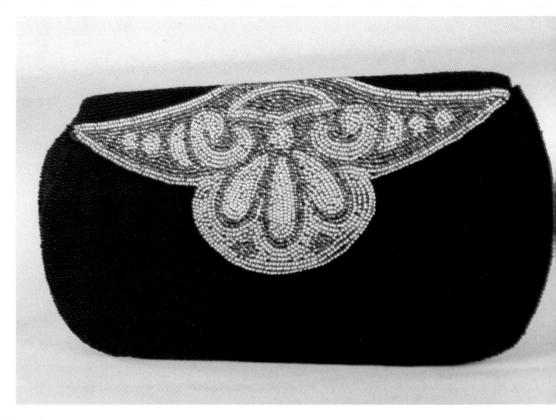

Ca. 1930 small, clutch style pocketbook, beaded all over with round, black glass beads; front flap decorated with round, silver glass beads, interspersed with swirls of round, white glass beads; lined with white silk; labeled Made in France.

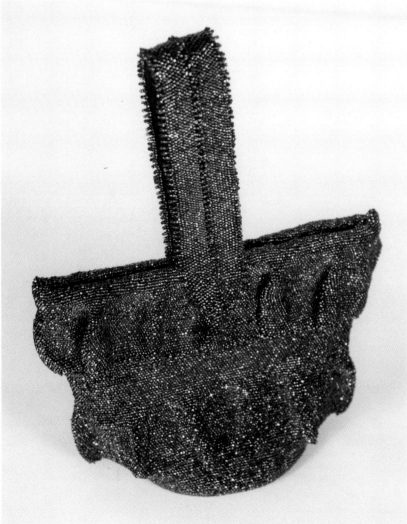

Ca. 1940 snap-clasp style pocketbook, beaded all over in charcoal gray, iridescent, round, glass beads; designed with gathers and tiers; lined with black taffeta.

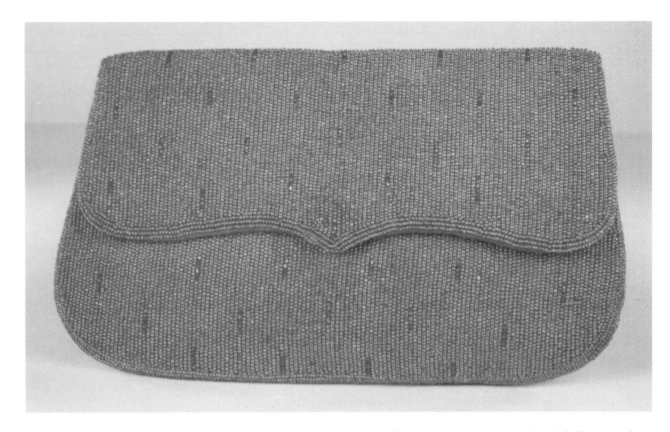

Ca. 1950 small clutch style pocketbook, beaded all over with opalescent red glass beads, interspersed with solid red glass beads; lined with ivory satin.

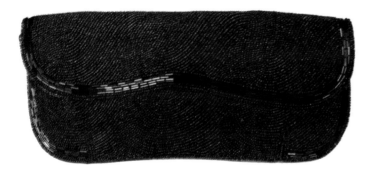

Ca. 1950 small clutch style pocketbook, beaded all over with round and bugle black glass beads; lined with black satin; labeled Made in France.

Ca. 1950 cylinder style pocketbook, beaded with round, black glass beads; black Lucite hinged top with a brass clasp and mirror inside the top; beaded handle; lined with black silk satin.

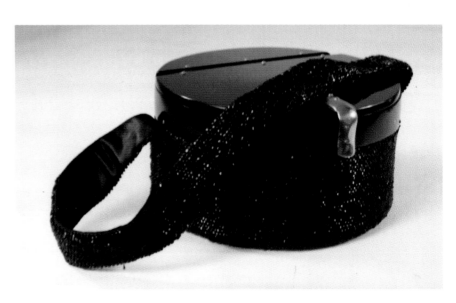

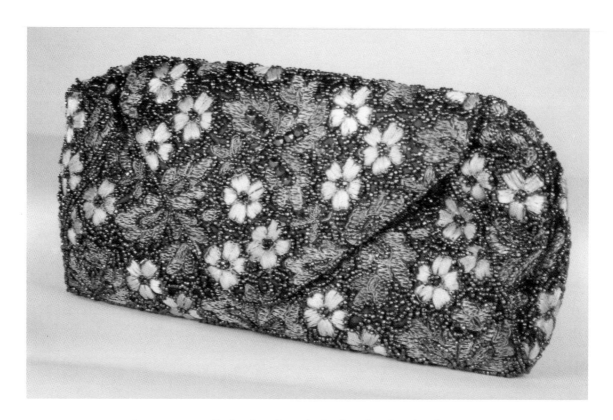

Ca. 1940 tan silk clutch style pocketbook embroidered and
beaded in a floral motif in shades of blue, lilac, white, and
pale green; lined with brown satin; labeled jemma "EV'RY
BAG A JEM."

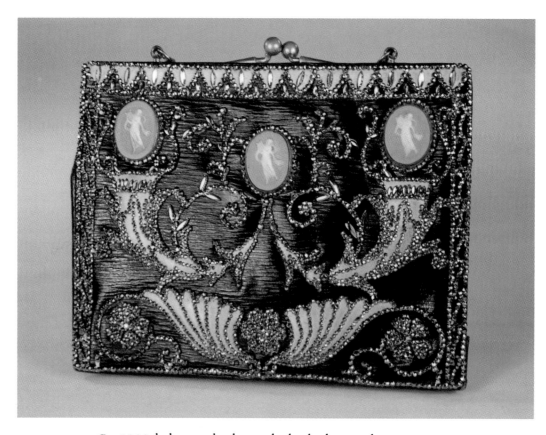

Ca. 1930 dark green leather pocketbook; decorated in a
classical motif with steel beads and Wedgewood blue
jasperware cameo ovals; chain handle. A very unusual
pocketbook! *Courtesy of Roslyn Herman.*

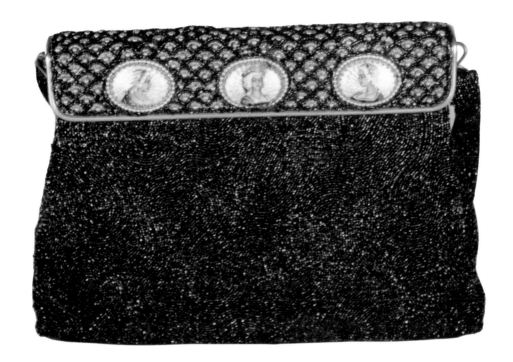

Ca. 1950 hinged clasp pocketbook beaded all over in swirls of
black, round glass beads; clasp decorated in black and gold
glass beads and beautifully enameled busts of ladies in 18th
century clothing; beaded handle. *Courtesy of Roslyn Herman*.

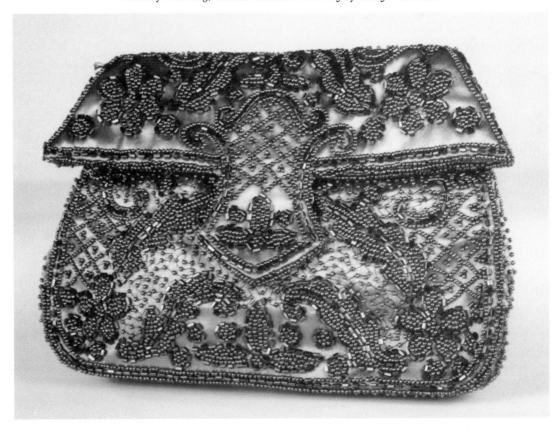

Ca. 1940 fold-over gray silk satin clutch pocketbook,
decorated front and back, in a floral motif, with charcoal
gray, round and bugle glass beads; lined with gray silk; labeled
Michel Swiss, 16 Rue De La Paix, Paris.

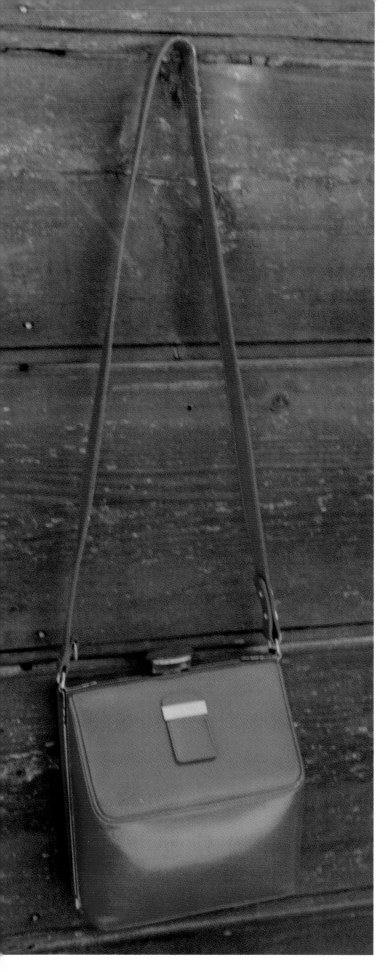

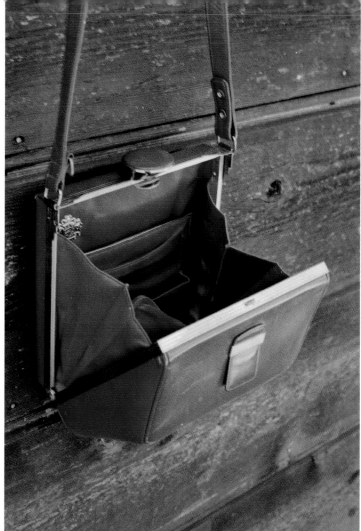

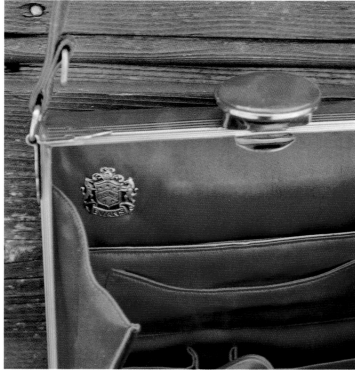

Ca. 1950 red leather pocketbook with a shoulder strap and a unique shape: brass frame, leather lined and detailed with Evans insignia. *Courtesy of Gemma Pomilio.*

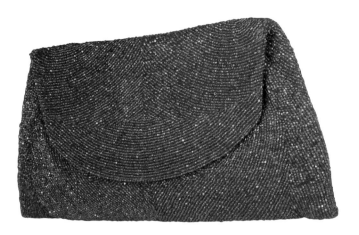

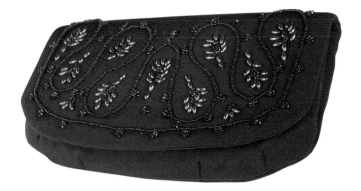

Ca. 1950 clutch style pocketbook, decorated all over in "swirls" of royal blue glass beads; some beads are iridescent; labeled Made in Belgium by Hand, Walborg.

Ca. 1950 navy blue silk clutch style pocketbook, decorated with rows of round, blue glass beads, and additional larger, rectangular, blue, glass beads.

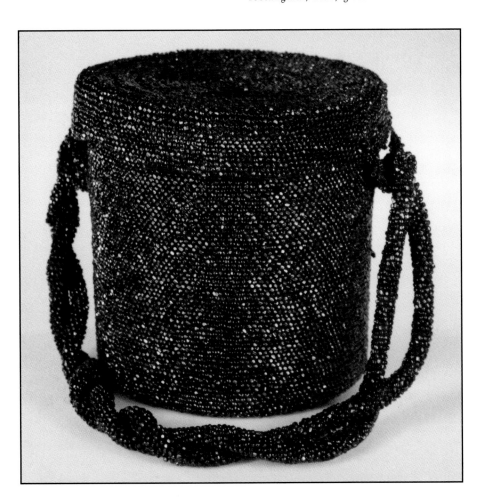

Ca. 1940 cylinder style pocketbook decorated all over with blue and purple iridescent, round, glass beads; top lifts up on braided handle which is also entirely beaded; mirror inside top.

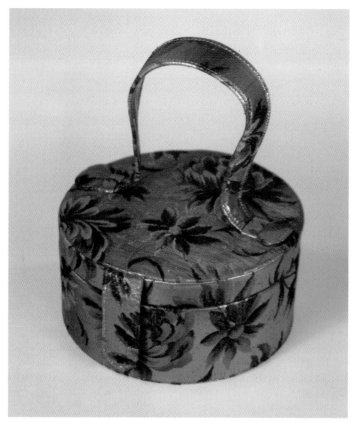

Ca. 1950 small cylinder pocketbook covered with gold brocade in a floral motif in shades of copper and dark brown; mirror inside top; snap closure; leather lined handle; lined with brown satin; labeled Lennox Bags.

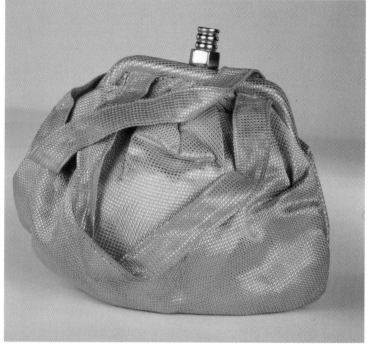

Ca. 1930 gold mesh pouch-style evening pocketbook; brass clasp; lined in ivory silk.

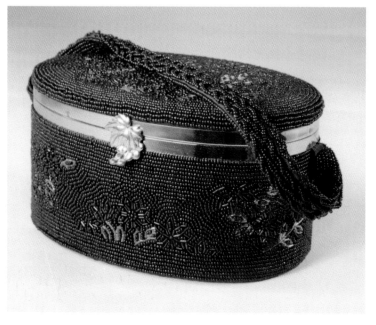

Ca. 1955 oval cylinder pocketbook beaded all over with round, brown glass beads interspersed with clear bugle beads; mirror inside top; beaded and braided handle; brass clasp in the shape of a leaf; lined with brown faille. An exceptional pocketbook!

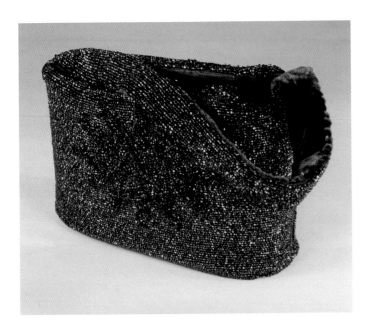

Ca. 1940 oval pocketbook decorated all over with round, copper, glass beads; lined with brown silk.

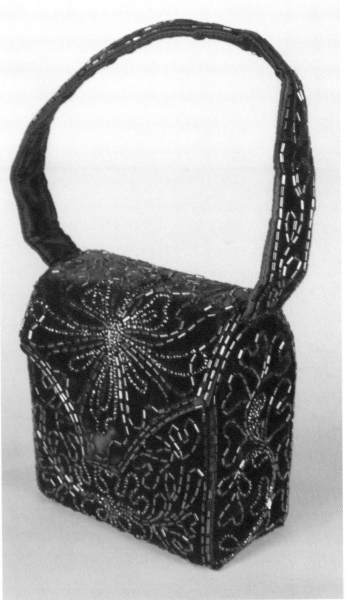

Ca. 1940 brown velvet, box-style pocketbook decorated with copper-colored, glass, bugle beads interspersed with copper-colored, round, glass beads; beaded handle in same material; lined in brown satin.

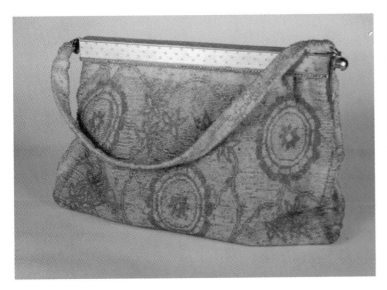

Ca. 1955 gold and silver beaded pocketbook; hinged clasp decorated with tiny rhinestones; ivory satin lining stamped in gold, designed for Saritzer & Fuhrmann Ltd.

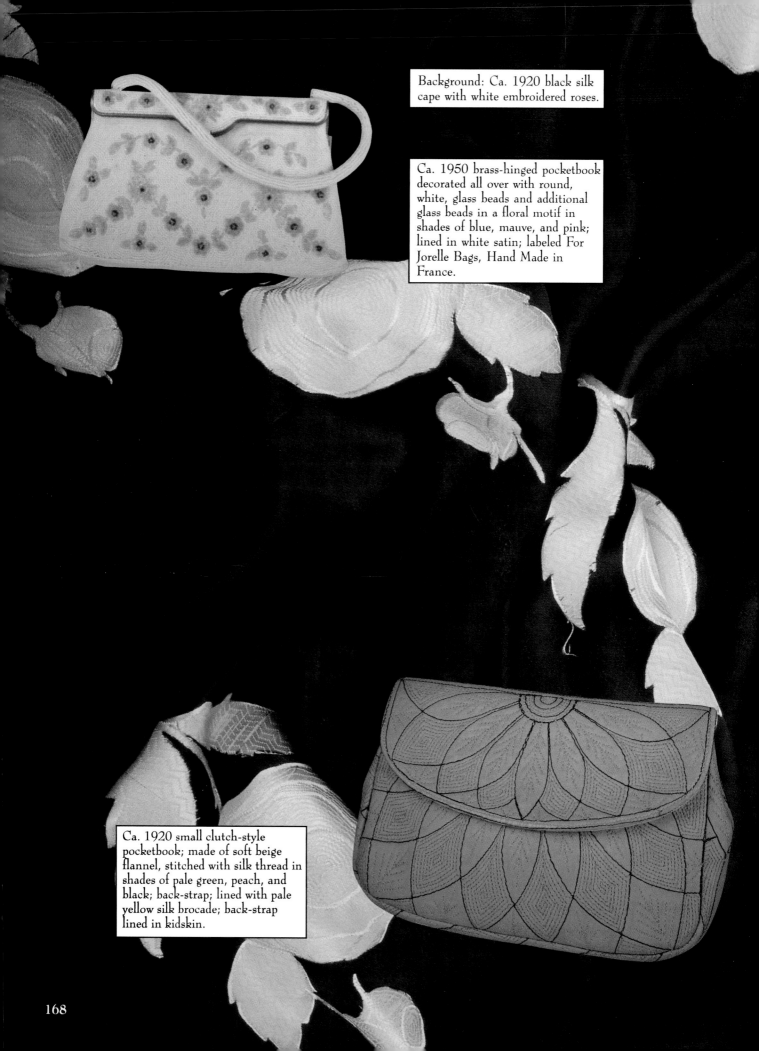

Background: Ca. 1920 black silk cape with white embroidered roses.

Ca. 1950 brass-hinged pocketbook decorated all over with round, white, glass beads and additional glass beads in a floral motif in shades of blue, mauve, and pink; lined in white satin; labeled For Jorelle Bags, Hand Made in France.

Ca. 1920 small clutch-style pocketbook; made of soft beige flannel, stitched with silk thread in shades of pale green, peach, and black; back-strap; lined with pale yellow silk brocade; back-strap lined in kidskin.

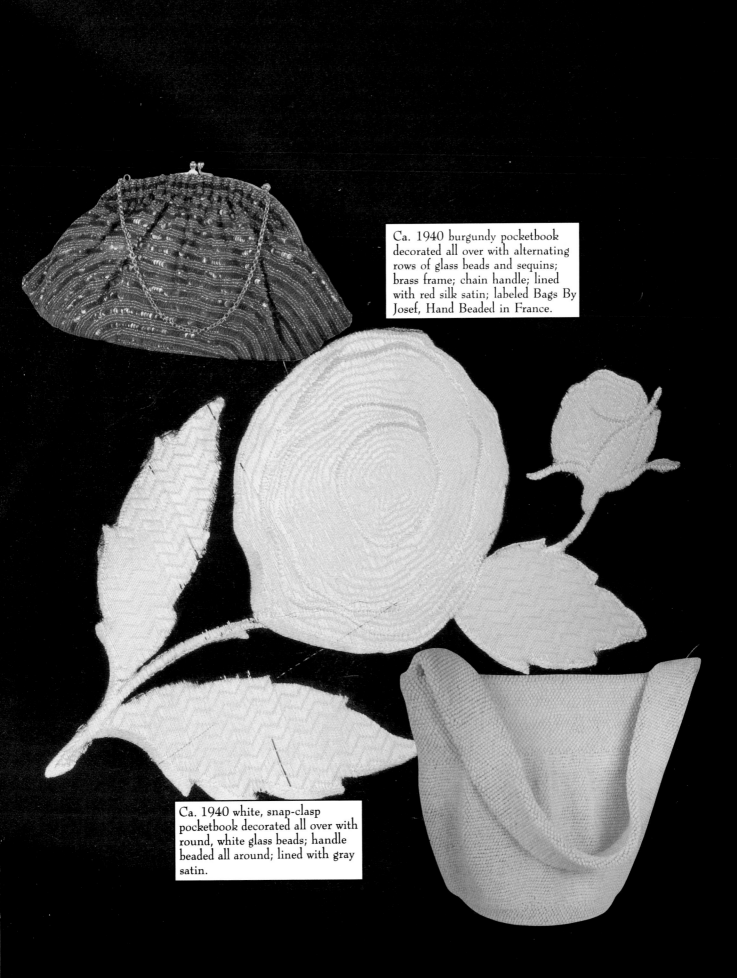

Ca. 1940 burgundy pocketbook decorated all over with alternating rows of glass beads and sequins; brass frame; chain handle; lined with red silk satin; labeled Bags By Josef, Hand Beaded in France.

Ca. 1940 white, snap-clasp pocketbook decorated all over with round, white glass beads; handle beaded all around; lined with gray satin.

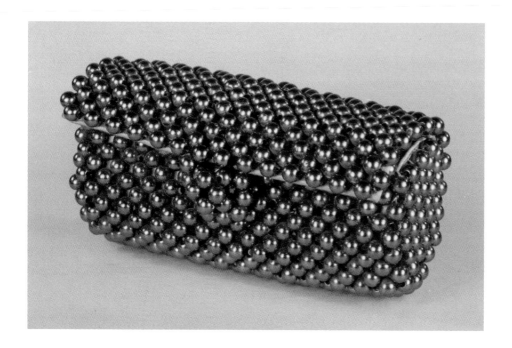

Ca. 1960 small clutch style pocketbook, beaded all over with gray synthetic pearls; lined with gray satin.

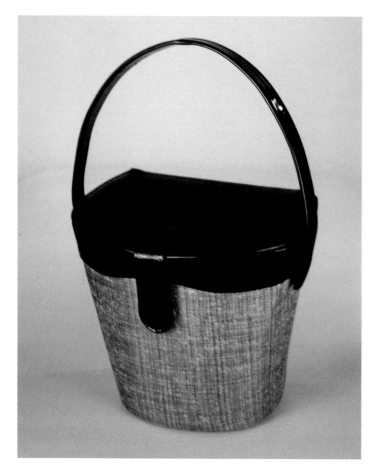

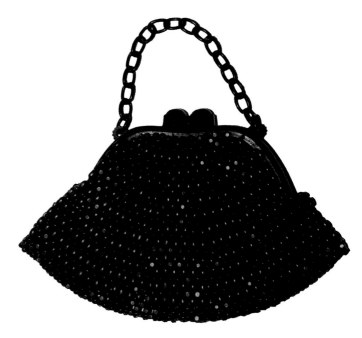

Ca. 1935 pocketbook made of black wooden beads with Bakelite frame and handle; lined with navy blue rayon faille.

Ca. 1950 cylinder pocketbook of black patent leather and gray fabric; patent leather strap and snap closure; lined with black taffeta.

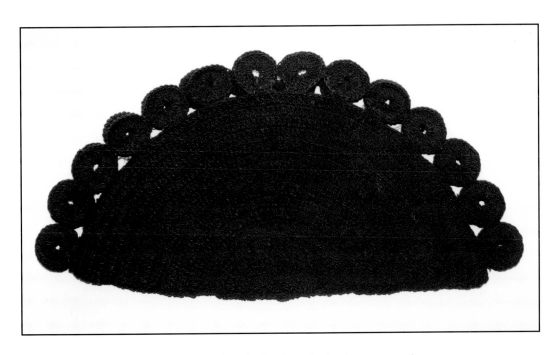

Ca. 1940 black, crocheted, clutch pocketbook constructed as a "folded circle" and edged with small, crocheted circles; zipper closure; lined in black faille.

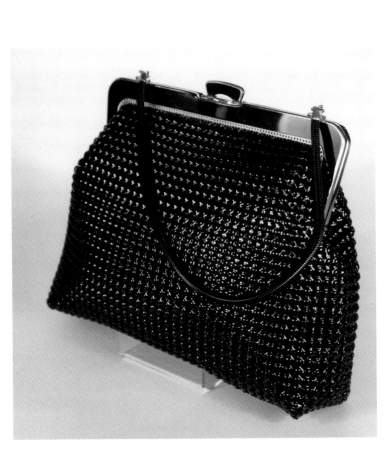

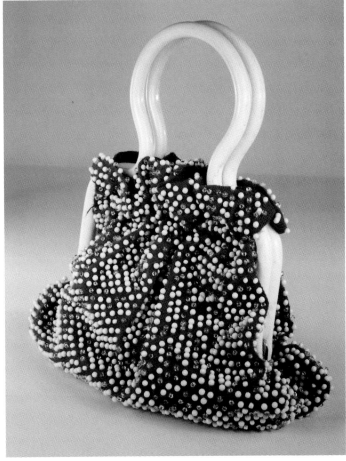

Ca. 1960 black enameled metal-mesh pocketbook on a gold and black enameled frame; metal handle; lined with black silk; labeled Oroton, Made in West Germany.

Ca. 1940 navy blue, cloth, pouch-style pocketbook beaded all over with white and clear plastic beads; white snap-hinged plastic frame with handles; small change purse inside with mirror, stamped Char-Mode Creations, N.Y.C.

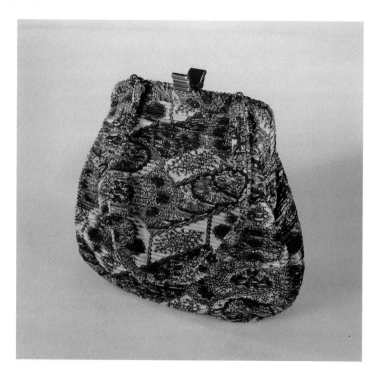

Ca. 1940 printed rayon evening pocketbook in a paisley design in shades of yellow, blue, red green, and white; brass clasp; lined with rust taffeta.

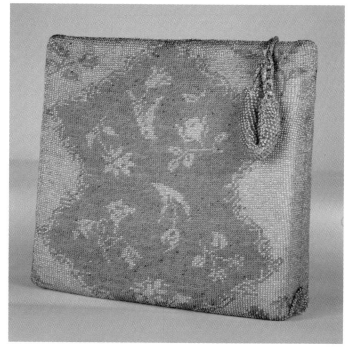

Ca. 1940 burgundy plastic, clutch-style pocketbook with a zipper closing on what stylistically appears to be the bottom of the pocketbook; decorated with small brass squares which are riveted through the plastic; lined with black taffeta. *Courtesy of David Sterner.*

Ca. 1940 square clutch style pocketbook, decorated all over in green and gold round, glass beads; zipper closure.

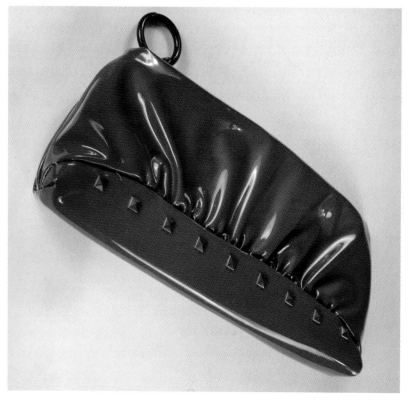

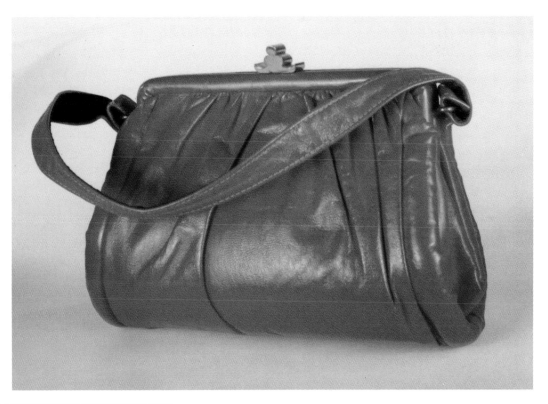

Ca. 1940 red leather pocketbook; leather covered frame; brass clasp; lined with black faille.

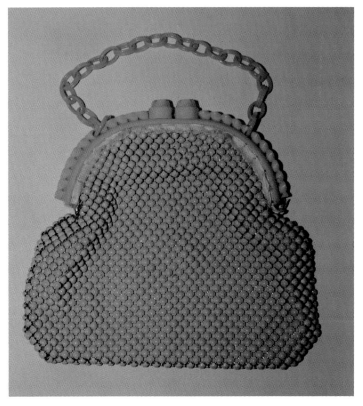

Ca. 1940 red velvet pocketbook, with a brass frame, and clasp detailed with red glass "stones;" same material handle; lined in peach colored satin.

Ca. 1930 ivory enameled metal-mesh pocketbook with an elaborate Bakelite frame and handle; lined with yellow silk taffeta.

173

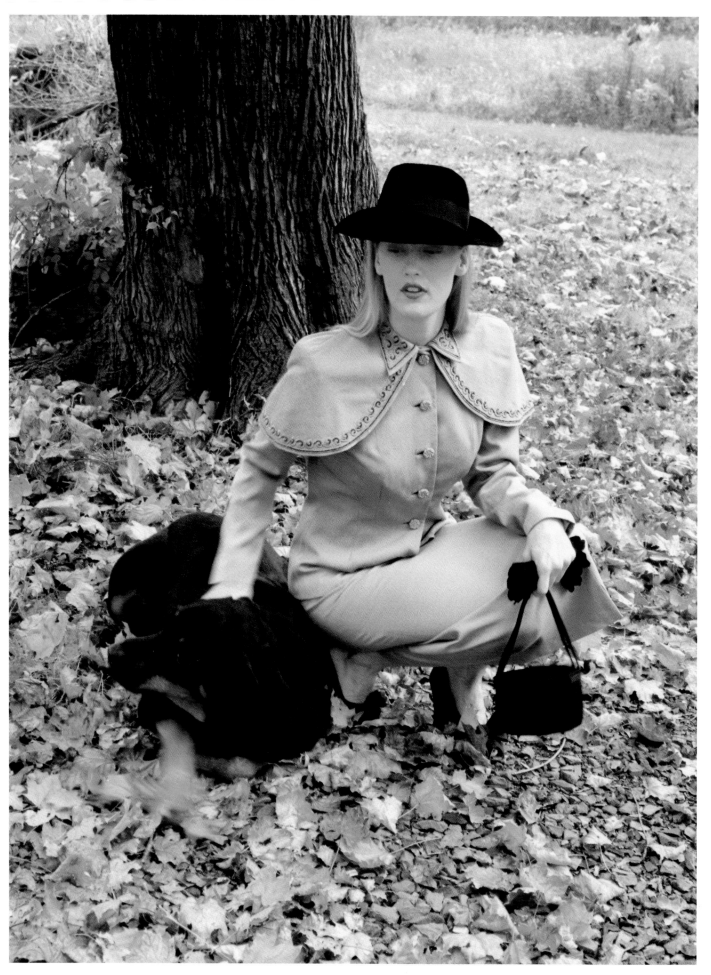

Chapter 5

Shoes

Shoes are made up of several parts; the *sole* or part under the foot, which includes the *heel,* the *vamp* or front part of the shoe, the *quarter* or back of the shoe, and the *shank* or portion under the instep. Shoes may be of the slip on variety, or may be closed with laces or buckles. Style and material relate to function. For example, shoes for evening wear tend to be made of more delicate materials than those made for day wear.

Vintage Style looks at wearable, fashionable shoes from the 1930s through the early 1960s. A few exceptional pairs of high-top lace-up, and button-up shoes from 1900 to 1910, are also pictured, to show a very functional style which has been reinterpreted by contemporary accessories' designers.

Terms that apply to many of the shoes of the 1930s and 1940s, apply to the shoes of the 1960s, and also to the shoes of today. For example, ankle-straps, shoes of the sandal-type, having a strap attached at the top of the heel which goes around the ankle, frequently made with a platform sole, were very popular in the 1930s and 1940s, but were revived in the 1960s and 1980s. The chunky heeled shoe, including the Harlow pump, a sabot-strap pump with a high chunky heel, named for Hollywood actress Jean Harlow in the 1920s, was widely copied throughout the 1960s and early 1970s, and has recently reappeared on the contemporary accessories scene. The *Mary Jane* style, a low heeled slipper with a blunt toe and single strap over the instep, buttoned or buckled at center or side, was named for shoes worn by the character Mary Jane in the comic strip *Buster Brown*, drawn by R. F. Outcault in the early 1900s. This simple style has been revised and reinterpreted throughout the decades since it first appeared. The platform pump, named after Carmen Miranda, a popular movie star who wore the style in the 1930s and 1940s, became very popular in the late 1960s.

Ca. 1940 pale gray wool gabardine suit with an over-the-shoulder cape and covered and embroidered buttons, soutache and beading on the cape and collar; labeled Jean's, Providence (most likely a retail store). A beautiful suit in terms of detailing and structure. *Modeled by Marcie Behanna, with Dallas.*

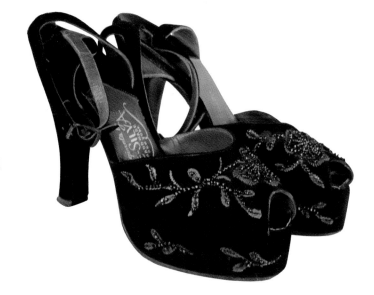

Ca. 1945 black, suede pumps with ankle-strap, open-toe, and high platform, embroidered and beaded on the toe, the heel, and the platform; stamped Originals of De-Silva, Hand Made, New York, and Metro Shoe Company, Inc., Fine Footwear. These shoes belonged to Gracie Boyajian Young who was the first Miss Atlantic City, New Jersey (Queen's Court, 1921).

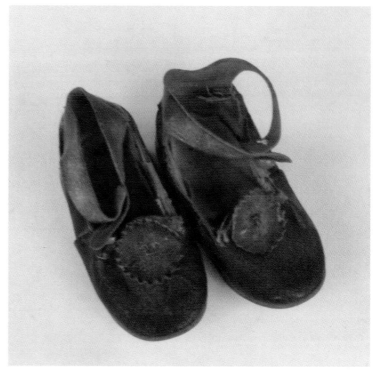

Ca. 1880 brown, leather, "Mary Jane" shoes for a very little girl.

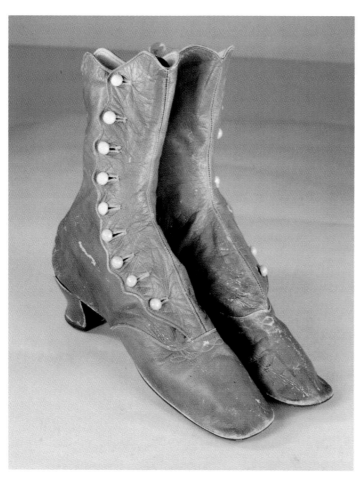

Ca. 1880 blue kidskin high-button shoes, with white glass buttons and "scalloped" tops; lined with white linen and kidskin; very likely custom made for a young girl; heel may best be described as a "baby Louis." My favorite shelf shoes!

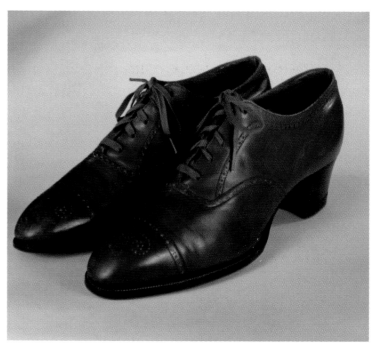

Ca. 1910 brown leather, low-heeled, lace-up shoes stamped in gold on the inside Strawbridge & Clothier, Philadelphia.

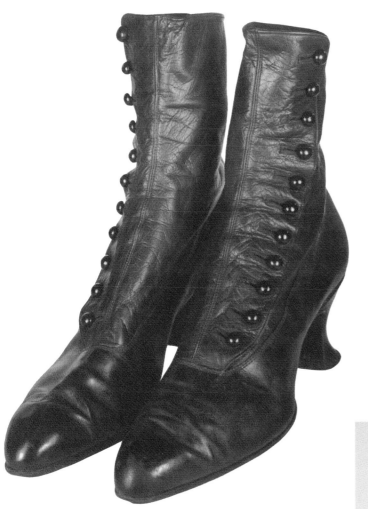

Ca. 1890 black, leather and kidskin, high-button shoes stamped on the inside Frank Brothers, Fifth Avenue, New York.

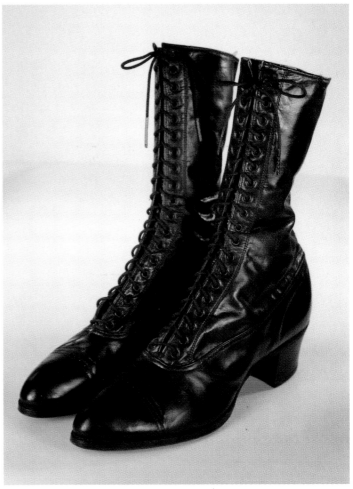

Ca. 1910 black, leather, high, lace-up shoes lined with ivory cotton twill.

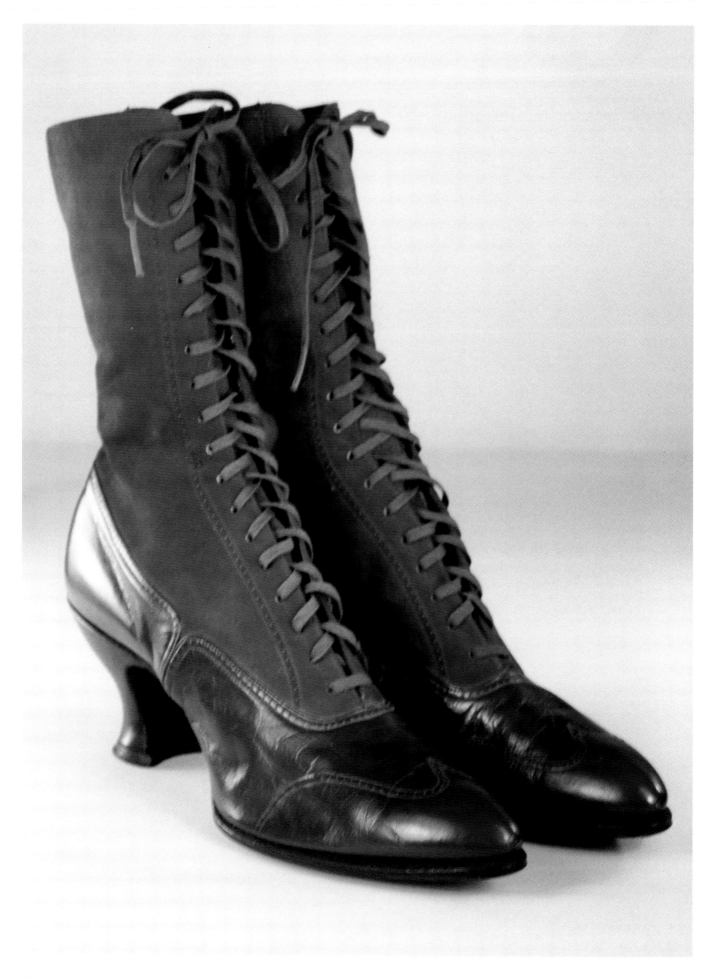

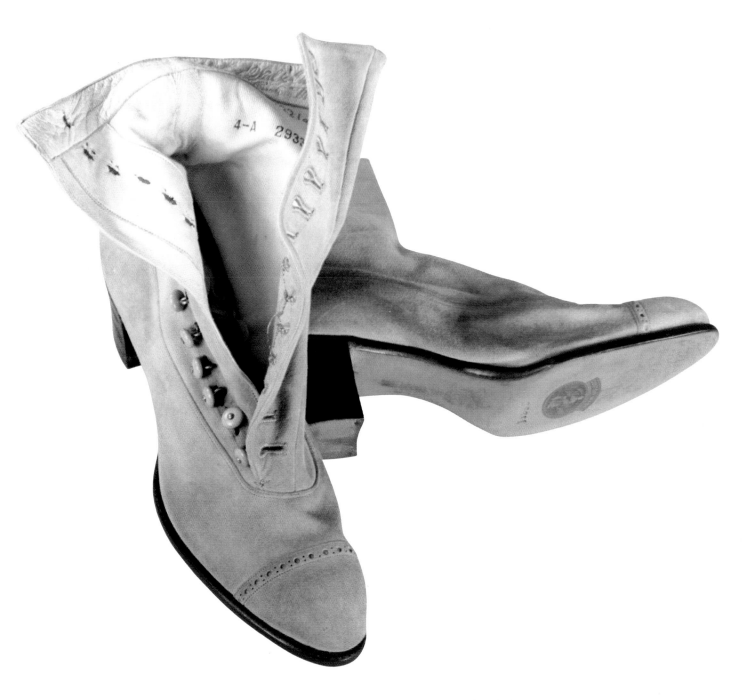

Ca. 1900 pale gray, suede, high, button shoes lined with fine
cotton twill and kidskin; stamped in gold inside the top Walk
Over, Custom Made.

Ca. 1900 burgundy suede and
leather, high, lace-up shoes
stamped inside the top Sorosis,
Reg. U.S. Pat. Off.

One store in America, F. W. Woolworth Company, has a shoe named after it, that has been entered in the permanent collection of the Metropolitan Museum of Art Costume Collection. The shoe, the *Woolworth*, also called the *landlady* shoe, has been sold in the millions by the Woolworth stores for over fifty years. It is made of cotton canvas in sandal style, in red, navy, paisley, black, or white.

The accessories' designer has always had the same dilemma--designing shoes that are salable, stylish, comfortable, durable, and at the same time appropriate for a myriad of occasions, activities, and seasons.

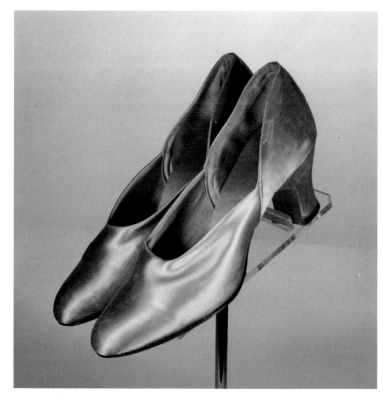

Ca. 1920 blue, silk, satin pumps.

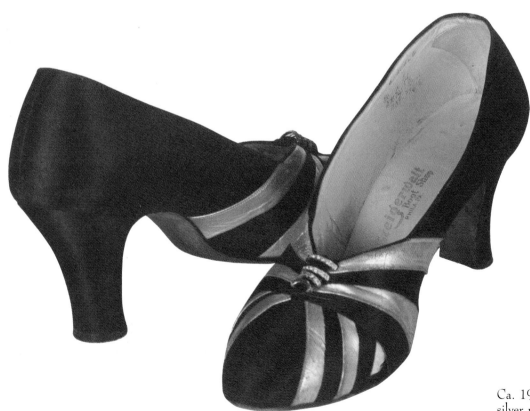

Ca. 1925 black silk, satin and silver pumps stamped inside Steigerwalt Boot Shop, PHILA. PA.

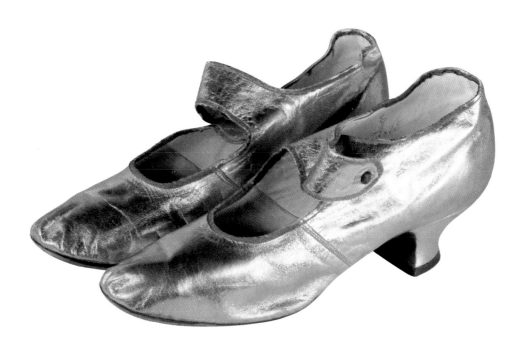

Ca. 1920 gold kidskin "Mary Jane" style pumps lined with white kidskin; found with newspaper dated 1925 in each shoe.

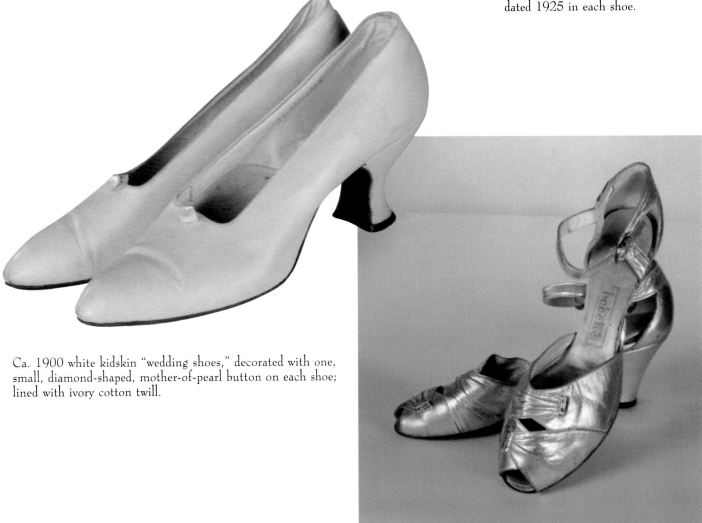

Ca. 1900 white kidskin "wedding shoes," decorated with one, small, diamond-shaped, mother-of-pearl button on each shoe; lined with ivory cotton twill.

Ca. 1930 silver, kid, open-toe pumps stamped babe.

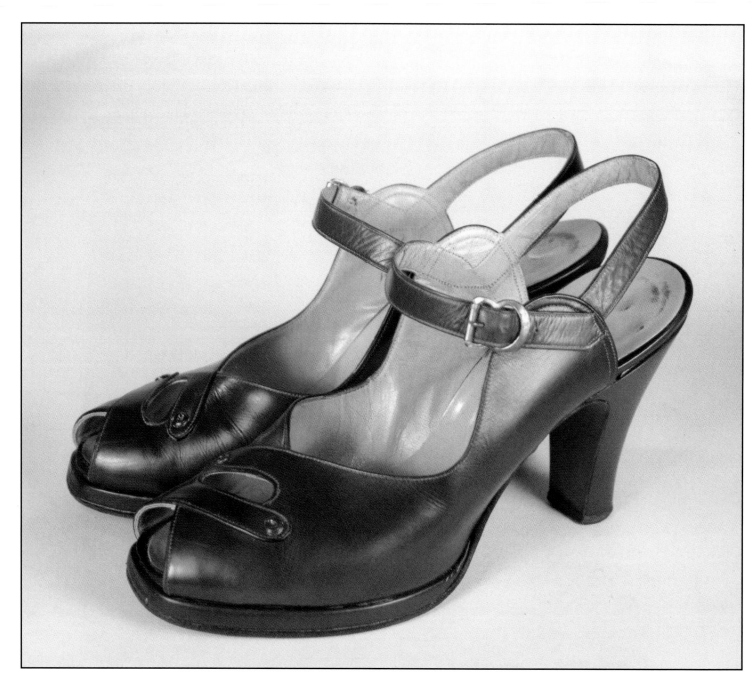

Ca. 1940 green leather, ankle-strap, open-toe, low platform
pumps.

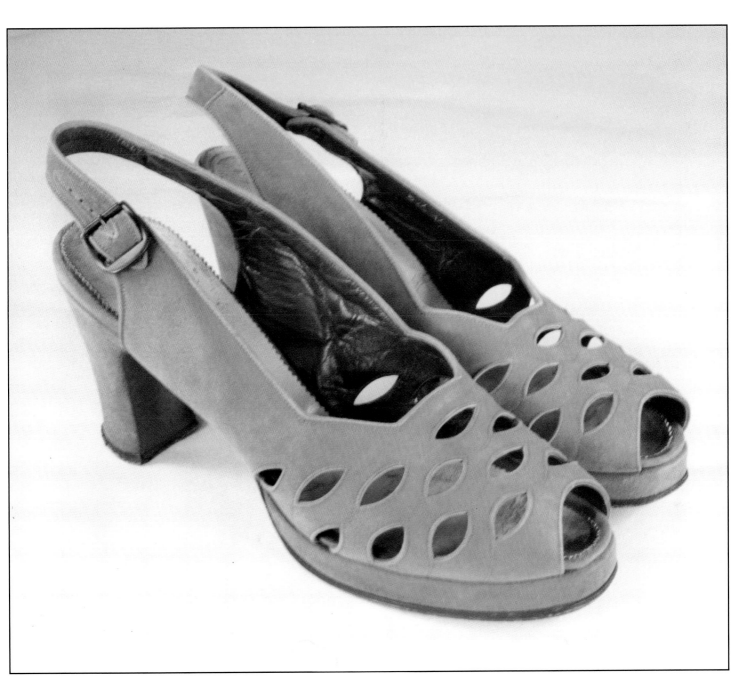

Ca. 1945 green, suede, sling-back, open-toe, low-platform pumps stamped Steigerwalt Boot Shop, Chestnut St., PHILA., PA. *Courtesy of the Drexel Historic Costume Collection.*

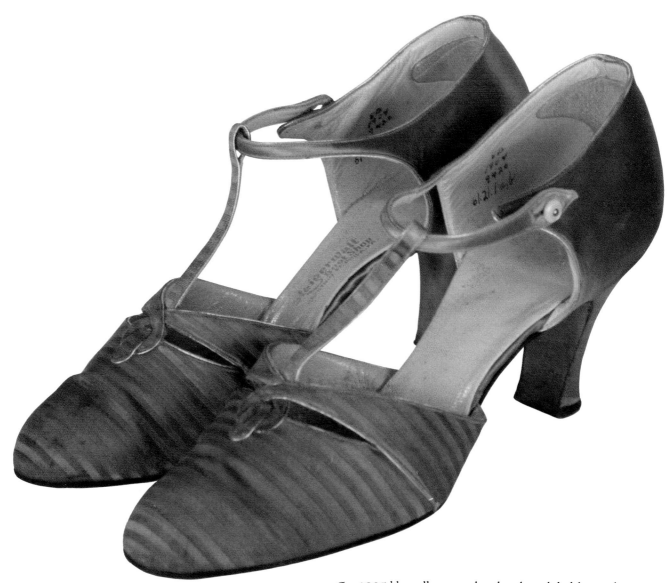

Ca. 1925 blue silk pumps lined with pink kidskin and stamped Daniel Green, Reg. U. S. Pat. Off., Philadelphia.

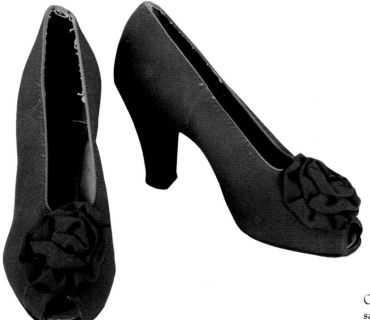

Ca. 1940 purple, cotton twill, open-toe pumps decorated with same fabric rosettes on the toes. *Courtesy of the Drexel Historic Costume Collection.*

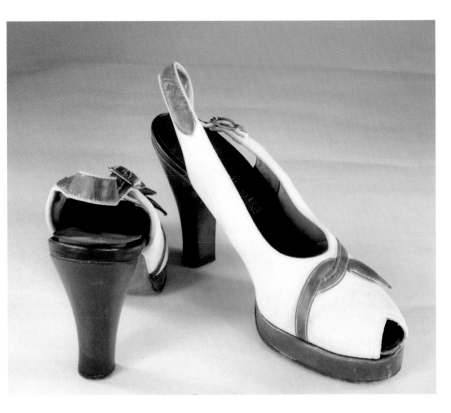

Ca. 1945 green leather and white suede, sling-back, open-toe, low-platform pumps stamped Valley Shoes, Bonwit Teller, Philadelphia. *Courtesy of the Drexel Historic Costume Collection.*

Ca. 1925 black silk, satin pumps with rhinestone-decorated heels; silk labeled Wise Shoe For Every Occasion.

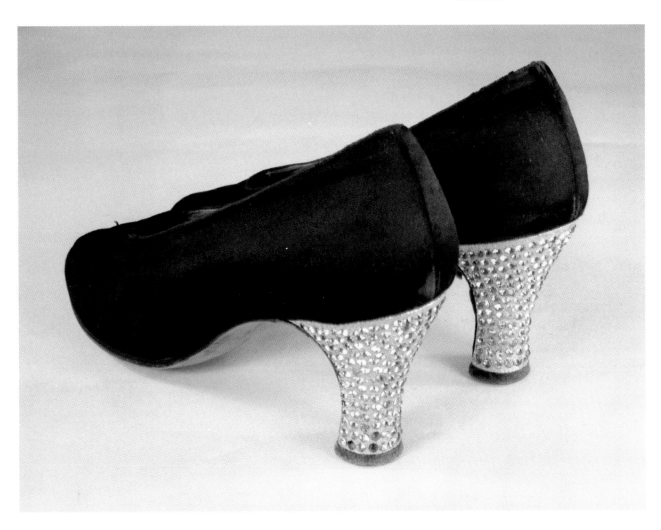

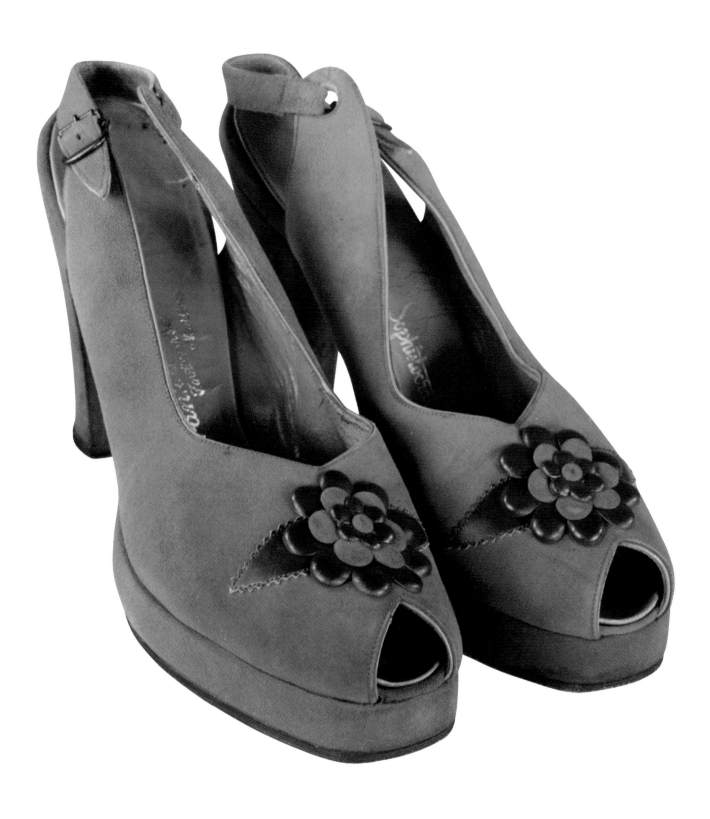

Ca. 1945 tan suede, open-toe, sling-back, low-platform pumps decorated with brown leather and tan suede flowers; stamped Frank Brothers Footwear Inc., Chicago, New York, Sophistocrat. *Courtesy of the Drexel Historic Costume Collection.*

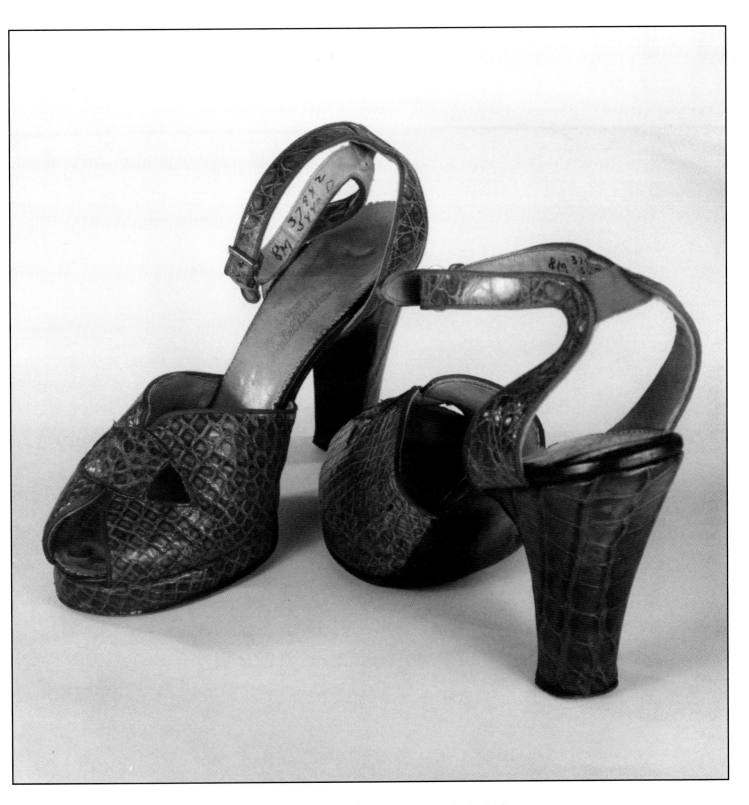

Ca. 1940 tan alligator, ankle-strap, open-toe, high-platform
pumps, stamped Made Exclusively for Gimbel Brothers.

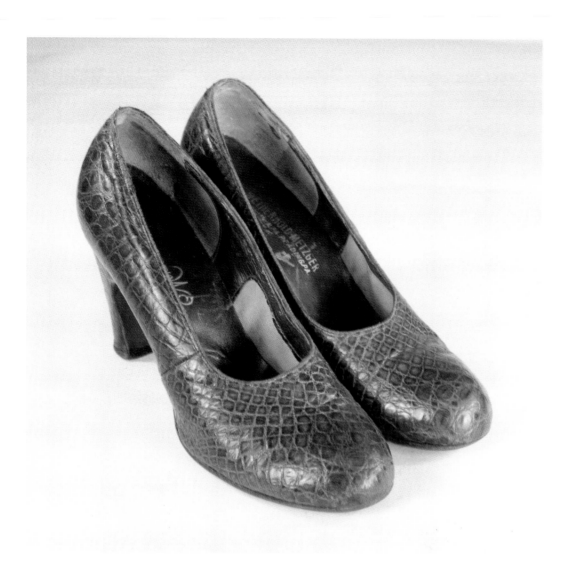

Ca. 1950 brown alligator pumps
stamped Menihan, Wetherhold-
Metzger, Allentown, Pa., Reading,
Pa.

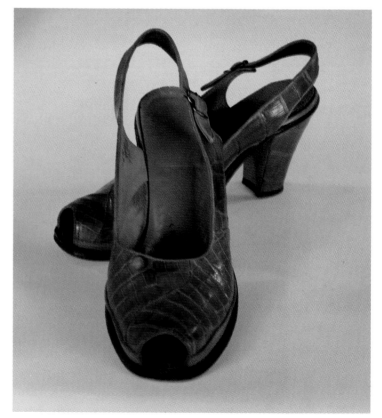

Ca. 1940 tan alligator, sling-back,
open-toe pumps.

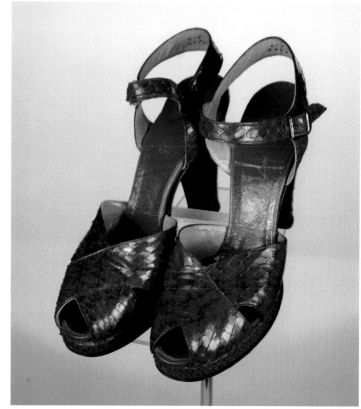

Ca. 1940 burgundy snakeskin, ankle-strap, low-platform pumps stamped Sky Lasts, John Wanamaker.

Ca. 1945 burgundy snakeskin and mesh, ankle-strap, open-toe, high-platform pumps stamped in gold, Custom Made. These shoes belonged to Gracie Boyajian Young who was the first Miss Atlantic City, New Jersey (Queen's Court, 1921).

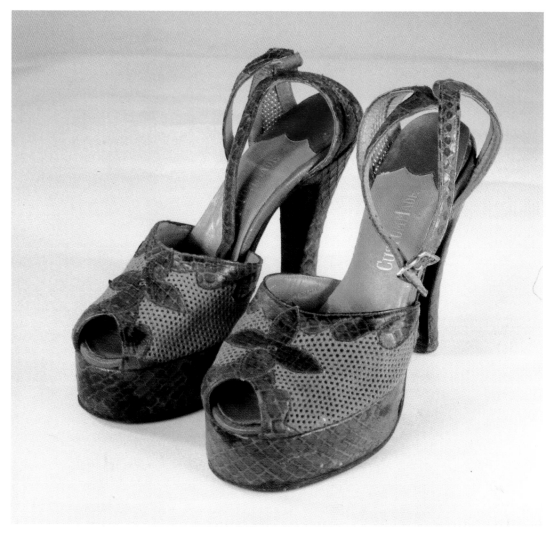

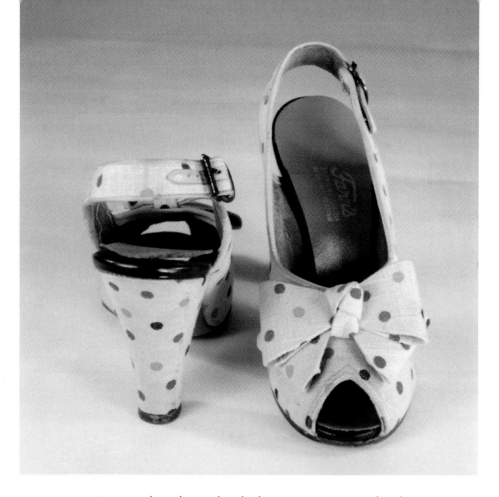

Ca. 1935 beige linen, sling-back, open-toe pumps with red, green, and orange dots; stamped Farr's, Allentown, Easton, Bethlehem, Reading. Described as "Minnie Mouse" shoes!

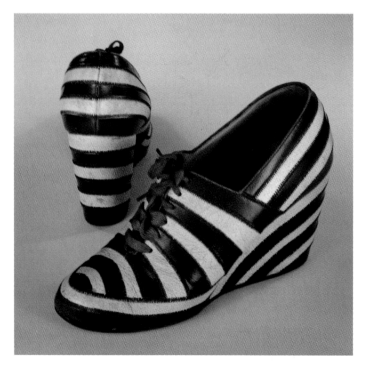

Ca. 1930 ivory and brown striped, wedge-heeled walking shoes; lace-up style; stamped Made By Premier, New York, Paris. These shoes belonged to Gracie Boyajian Young, who was the first Miss Atlantic City, New Jersey, (Queen's Court, 1921).

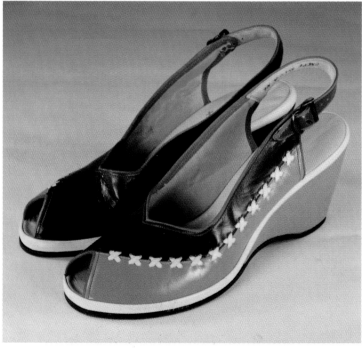

Ca. 1945 tan and dark brown leather, open-toe, sling-back, wedge-style shoes, decorated with cross-stitched leather in light beige; stamped floaters REG. By Turian, Charles Kushin, Oakland, Calif. *Courtesy of the Drexel Historic Costume Collection.*

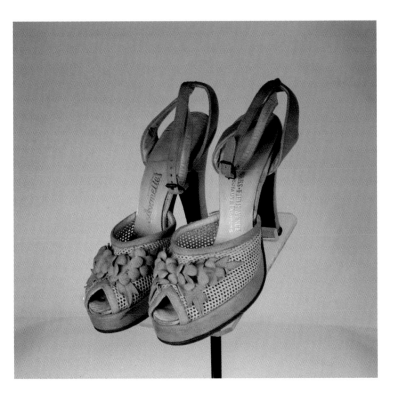

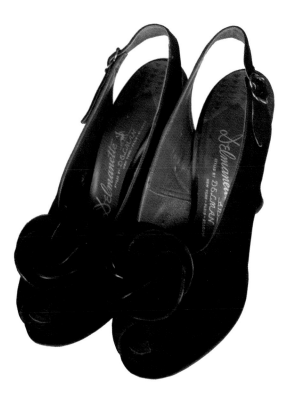

Ca. 1940 tan suede and mesh, ankle-strap, open-toe, low-platform shoes ,decorated with suede leaves and flowers; stamped Avonelles, Saks-Fifth Avenue, Debutante Fashions.

Ca. 1940 dark brown, suede, sling-back, open-toe, low-platform pumps; stamped in gold Delmanette, Styled By Delman, New York, Paris, St. Louis.

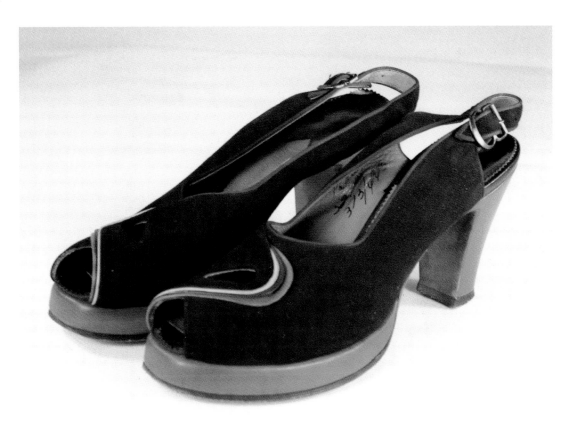

Ca. 1945 black suede, sling-back, open-toe, low-platform pumps, trimmed with burgundy and yellow leather; stamped Palter DeLiso Inc., New York City, W. H. Steigerwalt, PHILADELPHIA, PA. *Courtesy of the Drexel Historic Costume Collection.*

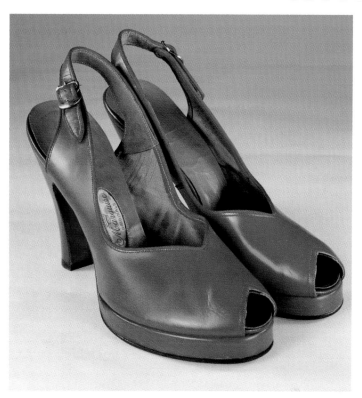

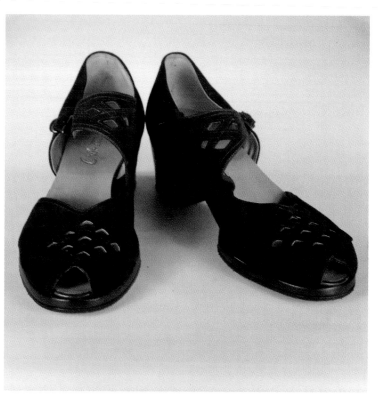

Ca. 1945 red leather, sling-back, open-toe, low-platform pumps labeled Marquise Originals. *Courtesy of the Drexel Historic Costume Collection.*

Ca. 1940 dark green suede, low-heeled, open-toe shoes with elaborate cut-outs; stamped Crick-etts.

Ca. 1940 black suede, ankle-strap, open-toe, high platform pumps.

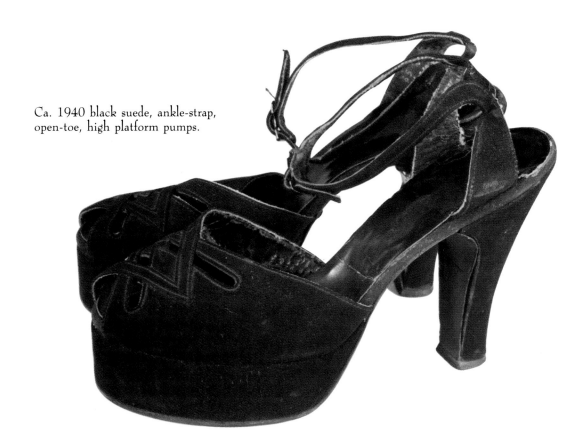

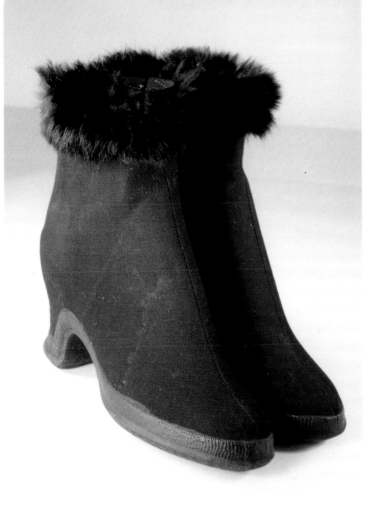

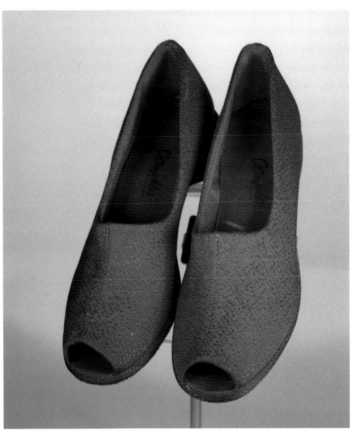

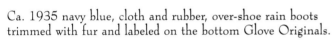
Ca. 1935 navy blue, cloth and rubber, over-shoe rain boots trimmed with fur and labeled on the bottom Glove Originals.

Ca. 1940 red, rayon slippers with leather soles; stamped Oomphies, Trade Mark.

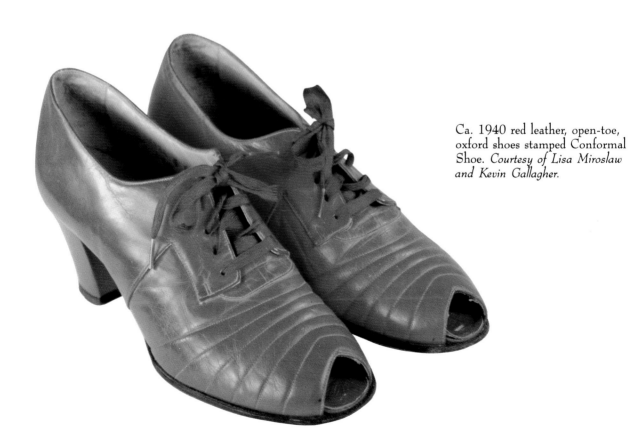

Ca. 1940 red leather, open-toe, oxford shoes stamped Conformal Shoe. *Courtesy of Lisa Miroslaw and Kevin Gallagher.*

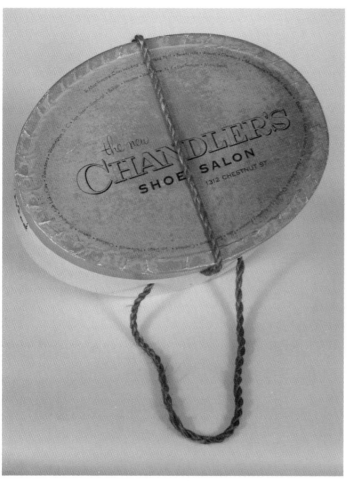

Ca. 1950 oval shoe box from Chandler's Shoe Salon, 1312 Chestnut Street in Philadelphia.

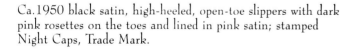

Ca.1950 black satin, high-heeled, open-toe slippers with dark pink rosettes on the toes and lined in pink satin; stamped Night Caps, Trade Mark.

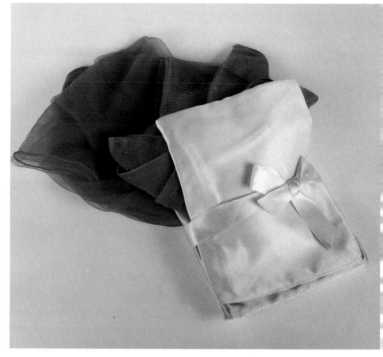

Ca. 1958 red and blue nylon stockings packed in a silk traveling pouch. Wearing stockings was a 1950s requirement. However, Donna Sigler tells how she avoided wearing nylons to church, and even fooled her mother, by using an eyebrow pencil to draw seams on the backs of her legs!

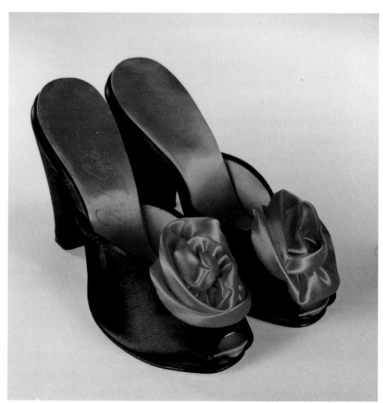

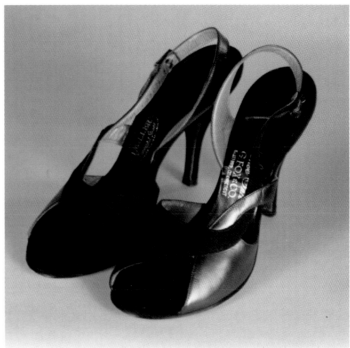

Ca. 1955 black suede and leather, spike-heeled evening sandals stamped I. Miller, Beautiful Shoes, G. Fox & Co., Hartford, Connecticut.

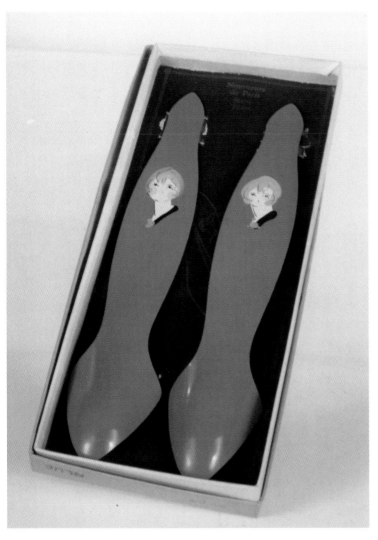

Ca. 1930 blue celluloid shoe trees, each painted with the face of a young woman.

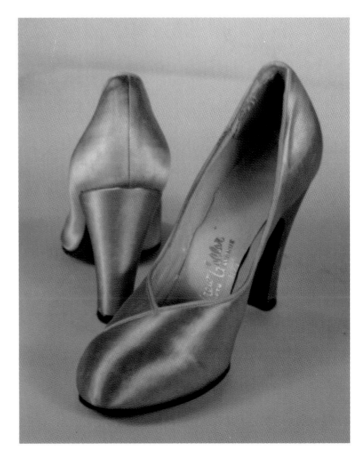

Ca. 1950 high-heeled, blue silk satin pumps lined with kidskin and stamped Andrew Geller, Fifth Avenue.

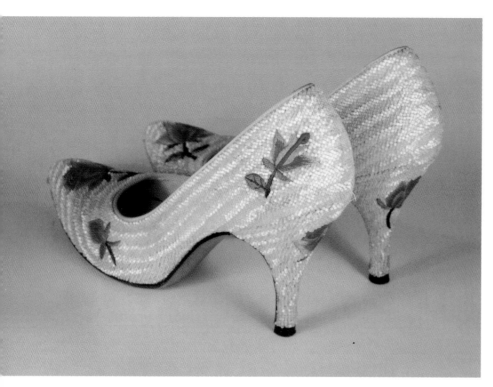

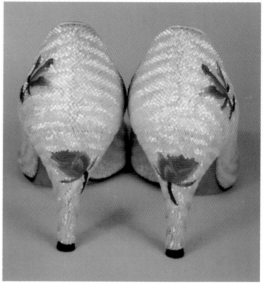

Ca. 1958 spike-heeled pumps beaded all over with opalescent white bugle beads, and further decorated with embroidered red roses. A spectacular pair of shoes! *Courtesy of the Drexel Historic Costume Collection.*

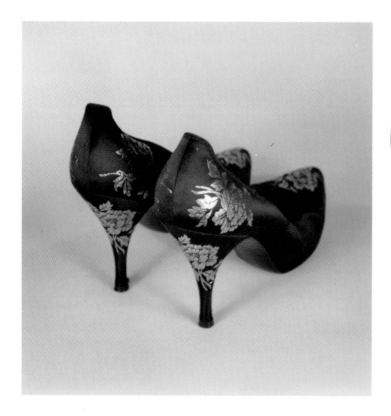

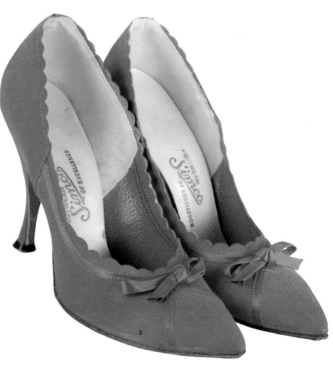

Ca. 1958 black and gold, silk brocade, spike-heeled pumps. *Courtesy of the Drexel Historic Costume Collection.*

Ca. 1955 bright red suede, spike-heeled pumps trimmed with satin bows; stamped Simco, Footwear of Excellence.

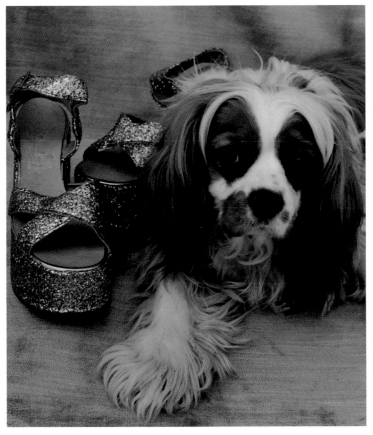

Honey goes for the gold!

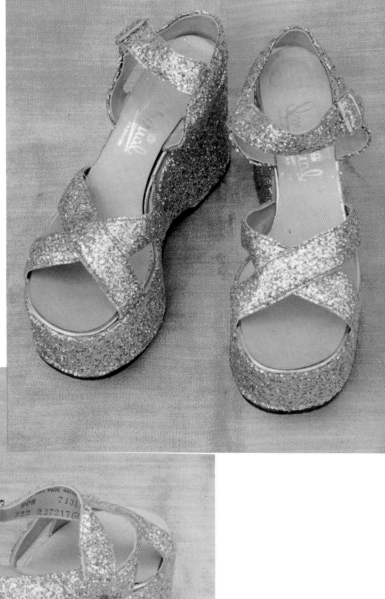

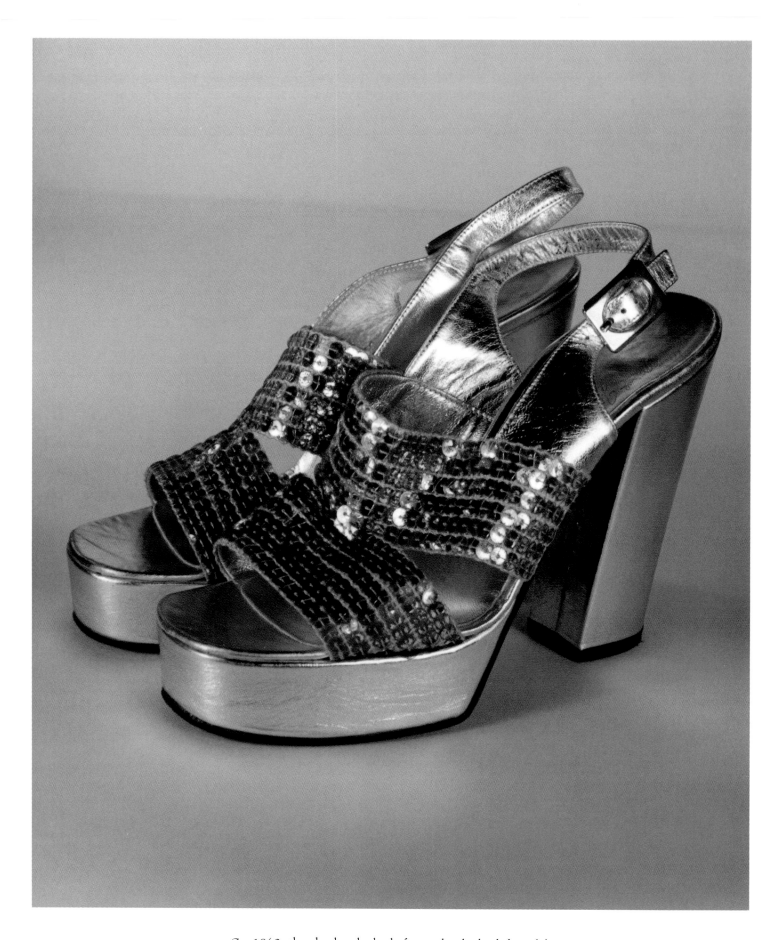

Ca. 1968 silver leather, high-platform, chunky-heeled sandals
decorated with silver sequins. *Courtesy of the Drexel Historic
Costume Collection.*

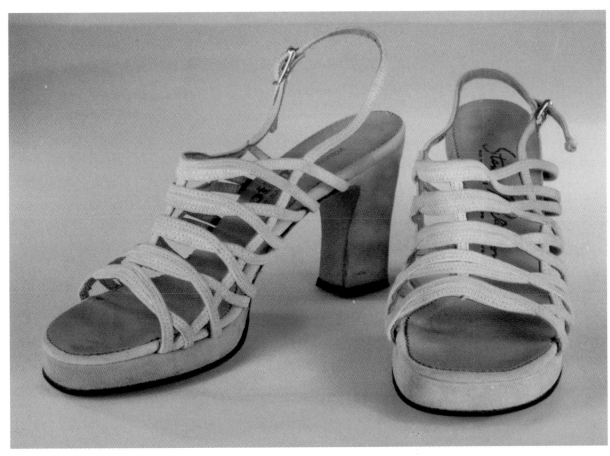

Ca. 1960 light blue suede, open-work sandals.

Ca. 1968 gold leather, high-platform, chunky-heeled sandals with criss-crossed, wide straps.

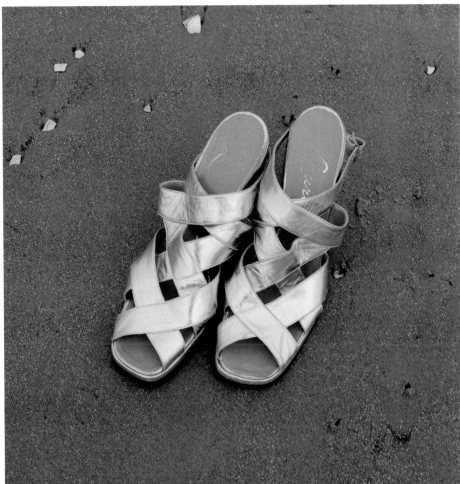

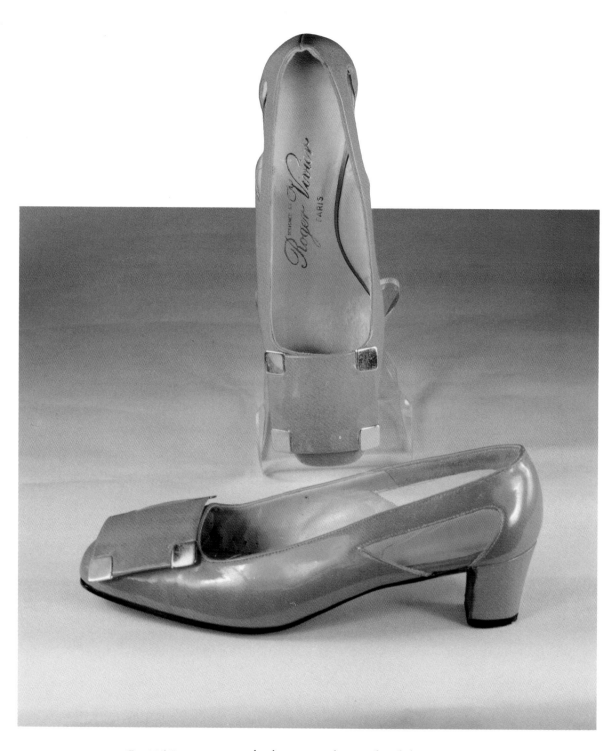

Ca. 1965 orange patent leather pumps decorated with brass-cornered, square buckles and open sides; stamped Designed by Roger Vivier, Paris, Saks Fifth Avenue. *Courtesy of Matthew Smith.*

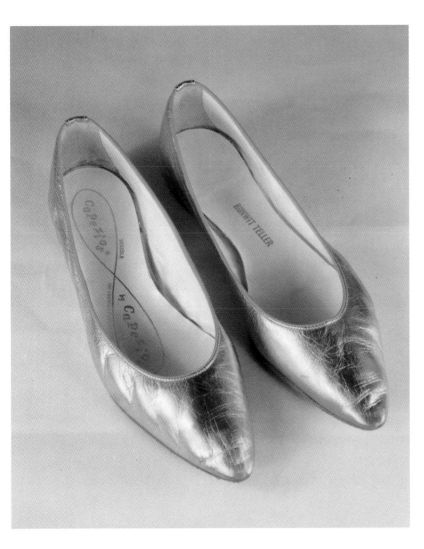

Ca. 1960 gold, leather, ballet flats lined with white kidskin and stamped Skeedle Capezios, by Capezio, The Dancer's Cobbler Since 1887. Purchased new by the author in 1960.

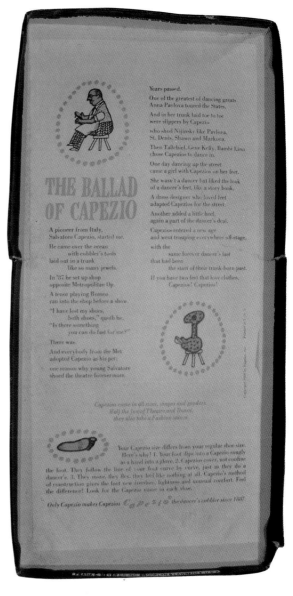

A Capezio box lid with the printed "Ballad of Capezio" which relates the story of Salvatore Capezio who came from Italy, in 1887, and opened a shop in New York City, opposite the Metropolitan Opera Company.

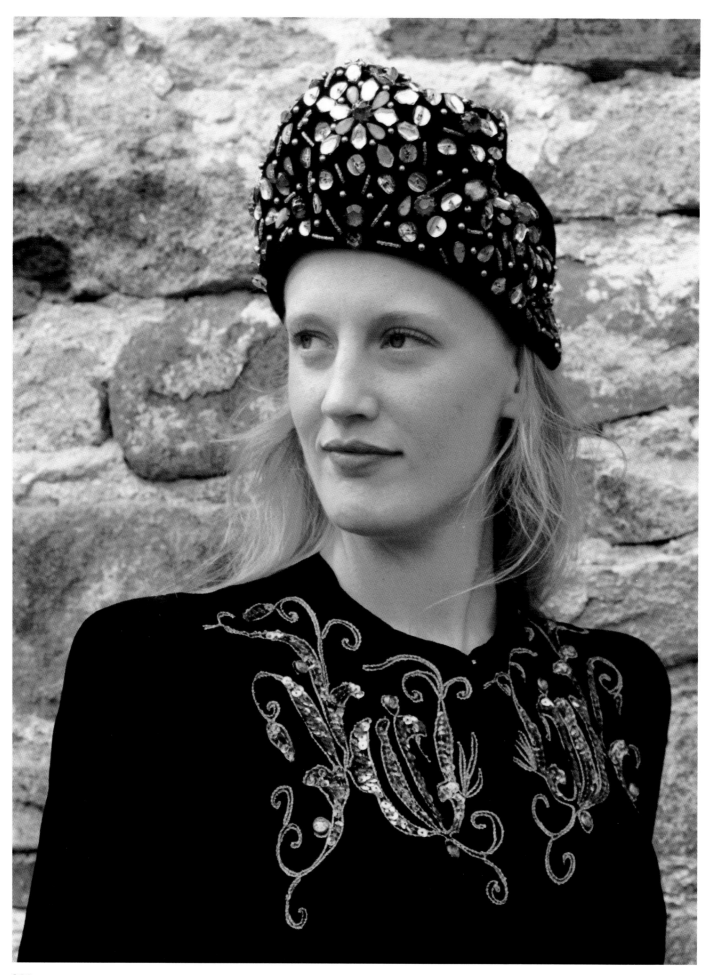

Chapter 6
Hats

There has been a renewed interest in millinery in recent years, but hair still seems to be making the pre-eminent fashion statement! Collectors of vintage hats defy the trends, looking for individuality and glamour. Women involved in the arts, theater, and even the more traditional fields, such as law, find in millinery an exciting image-maker.

The most difficult aspect of understanding vintage millinery is dating it. Since the styles from the late 19th to the early 20th centuries tend to be more difficult to locate, and more expensive to purchase, than later styles that are more abundant, it is important as a collector to have some idea of styles and dates.

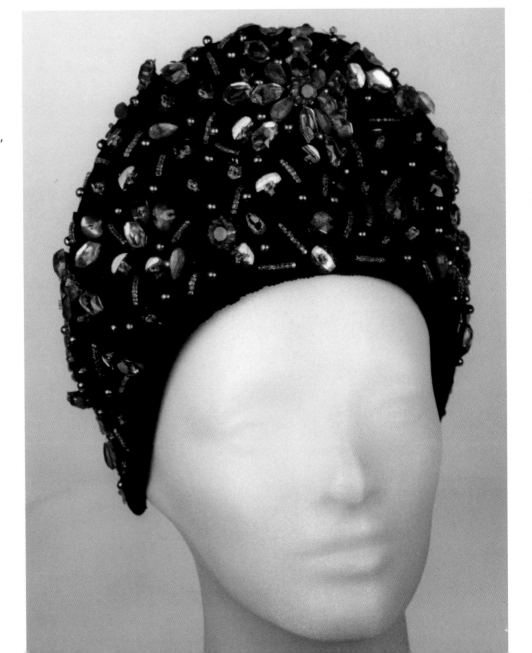

Ca. 1940 black, velvet, evening coat embroidered with gold thread and gold sequins and lined with ivory crepe; worn with a black felt hat of the same period which is decorated with colored rhinestones, sequins, and beads; hat labeled Leslie James, California. *Modeled by Marcie Behanna.*

Ca. 1940 black felt hat, elaborately decorated with beads, rhinestones, and sequins; labeled Leslie James, California.

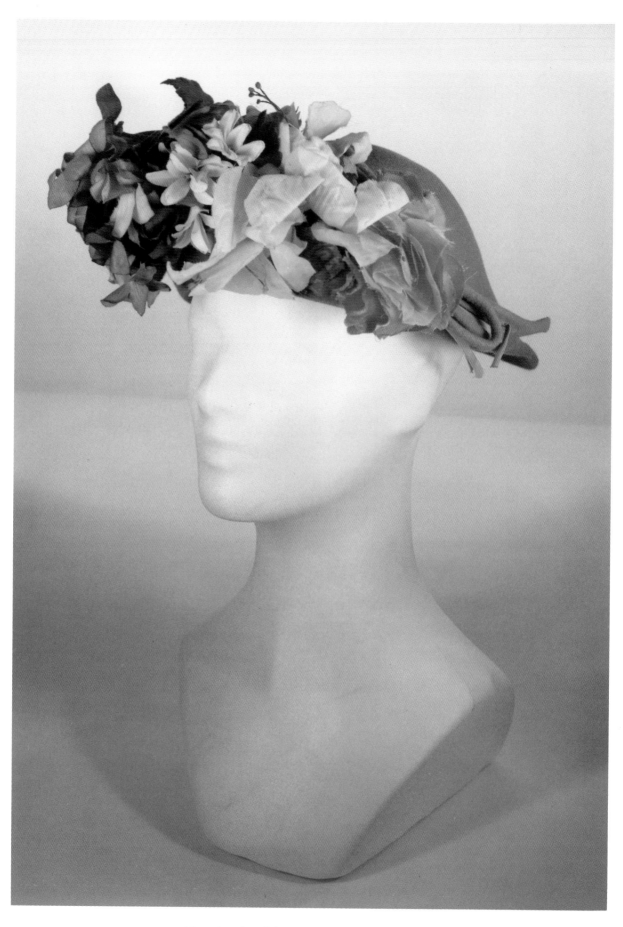

Ca. 1945 lilac velour hat elaborately trimmed with silk flowers;
labeled Lilly Daché.

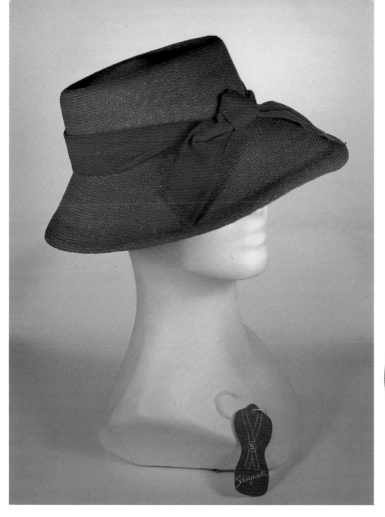

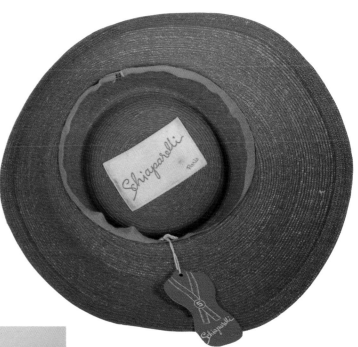

Ca. 1950 dyed red, wide-brimmed, straw hat, trimmed with a silk, grosgrain ribbon and labeled Schiaparelli, Paris; the original small, "shocking" pink, Schiaparelli, "dress form" tag hangs from the inside band.

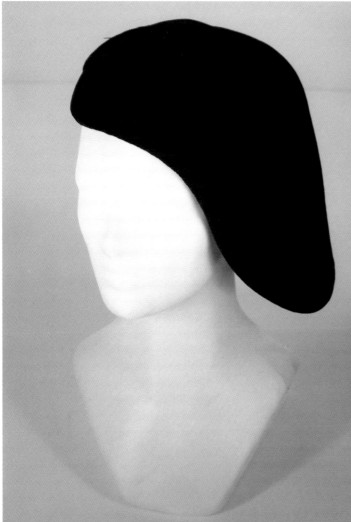

Ca. 1950 black, silk velvet, asymmetrical hat; labeled Sally Victor.

Ca. 1920 blue ostrich plume attached to a black, composition button specially designed for trimming millinery.

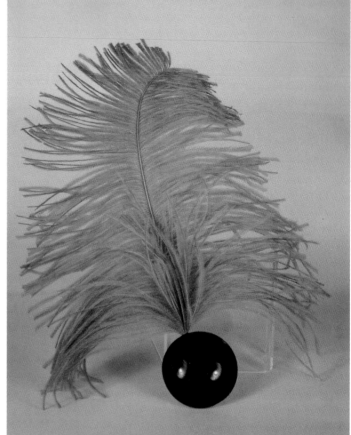

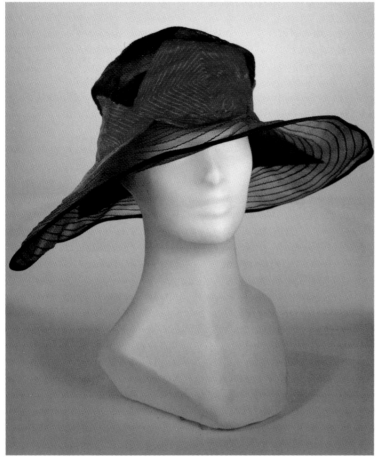

Ca. 1920 brown, horsehair hat trimmed with elaborately stitched tangerine silk velvet squares; labeled Philmont Hat.

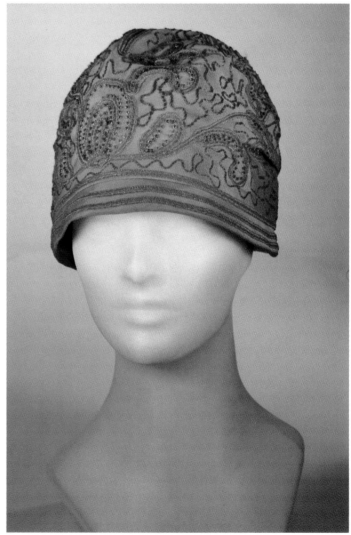

Ca. 1920 peach silk, faille cloche embroidered with silk thread and horsehair, and further decorated with round, clear, glass beads; lined with ivory silk.

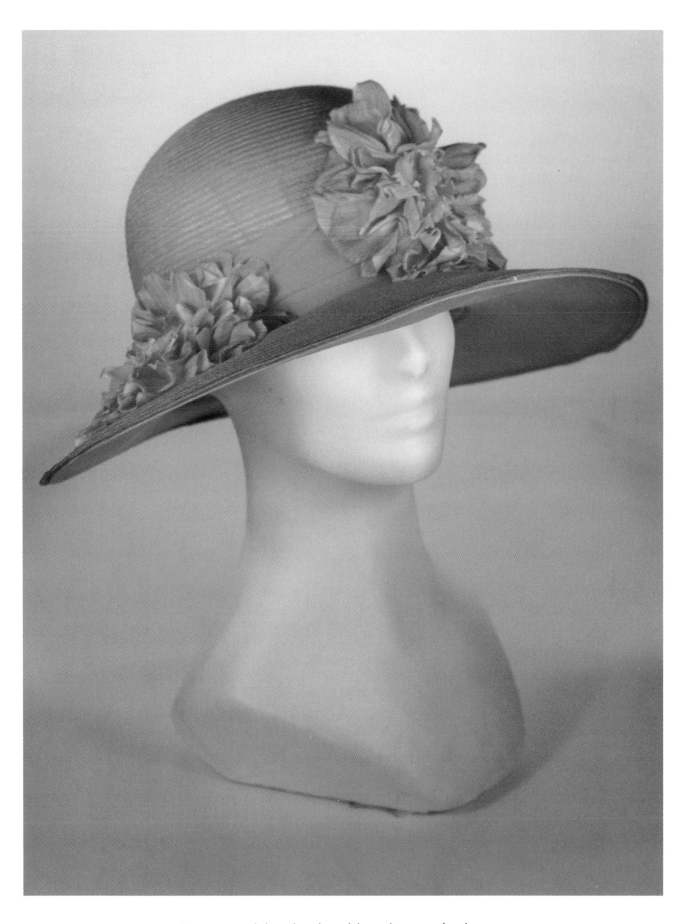

Ca. 1920 peach horsehair hat, elaborately trimmed with
peach chiffon and silk flowers; lined with ivory silk; labeled
John Wanamaker Modes, Philadelphia.

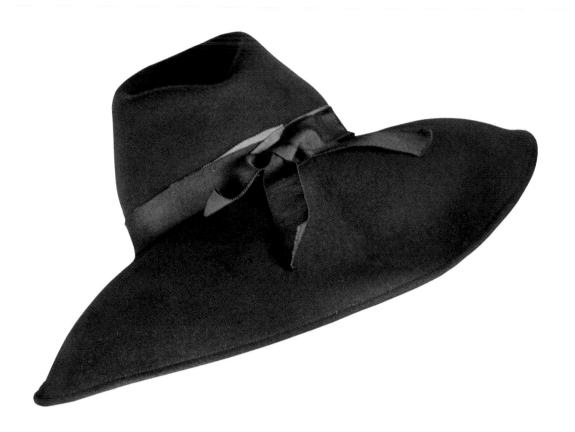

Ca. 1940 bright green felt fedora, trimmed with tan and green grosgrain ribbon.

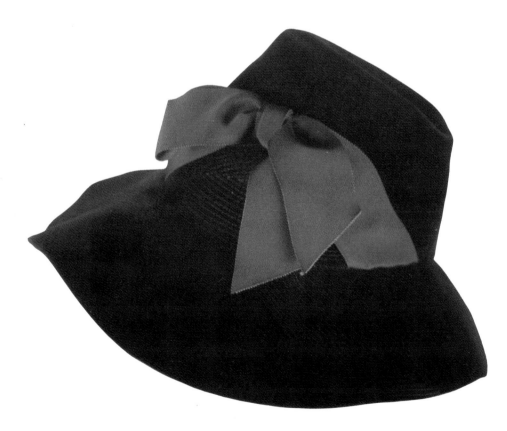

Ca. 1940 dark green velour fedora trimmed with a green grosgrain bow. A soft and beautifully designed hat!

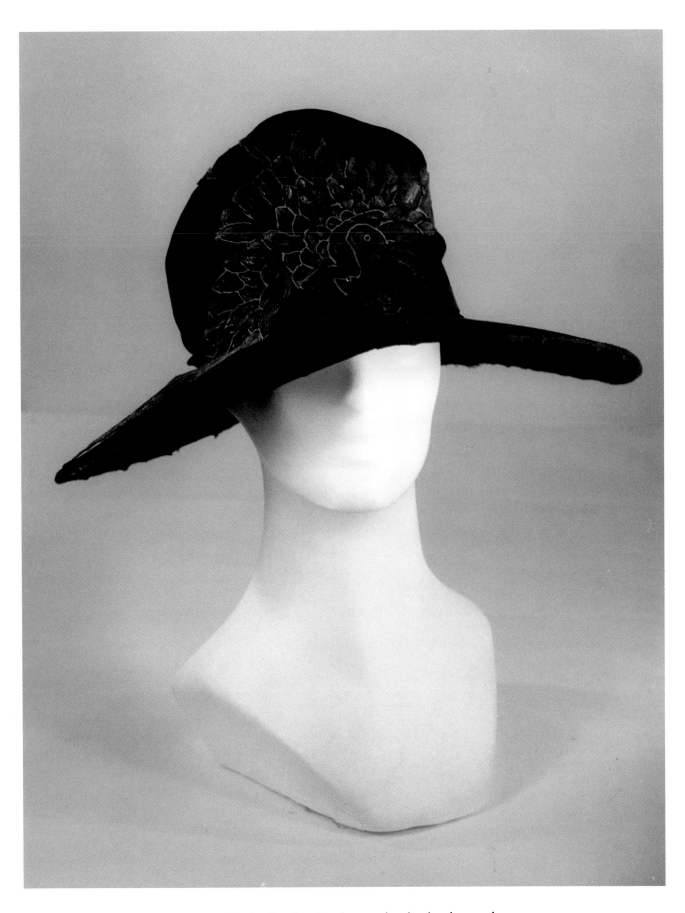

Ca. 1920 black silk velvet hat decorated with a hand-painted bird in shades of blue, green, red, and gold; lined with iridescent purple silk; labeled Gage Brothers, Chicago, New York, Paris; the original price tag inside is for $9.50.

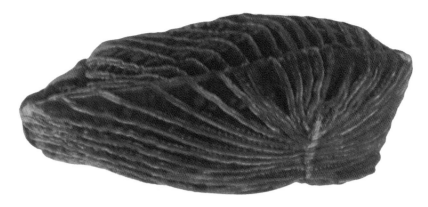

Ca. 1950 gathered and stitched, purple velvet hat.

In the foreground, ca. 1930, miniature Stetson, brown felt bowler hat, trimmed with lighter brown silk and with a leather, inside band; miniature Stetson hat box shown, for comparison, with a regular size women's hat box.

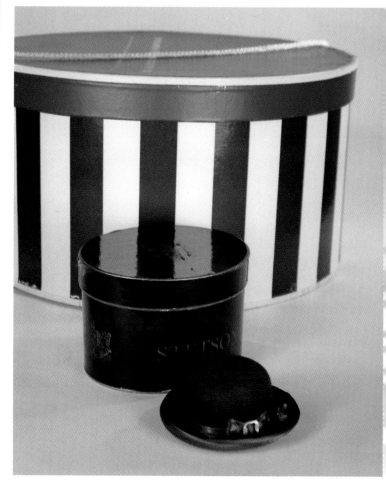

Ca. 1935 blue velour, pointed-crown hat with a blue and rose braided band and streamers. This design may have been inspired by the witch's hat in the movie *The Wizard of Oz*.

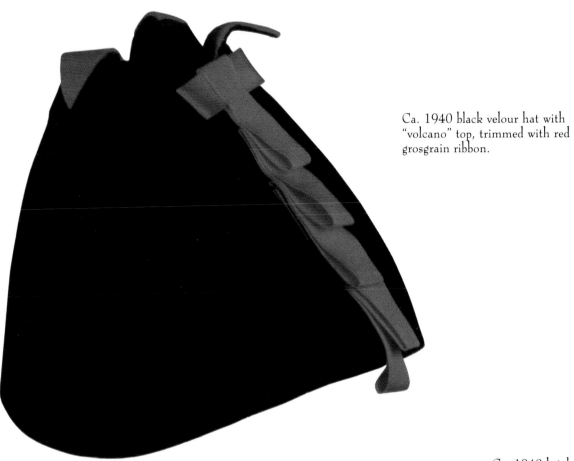

Ca. 1940 black velour hat with "volcano" top, trimmed with red grosgrain ribbon.

Ca. 1940 bright red velour hat, trimmed with the same material.

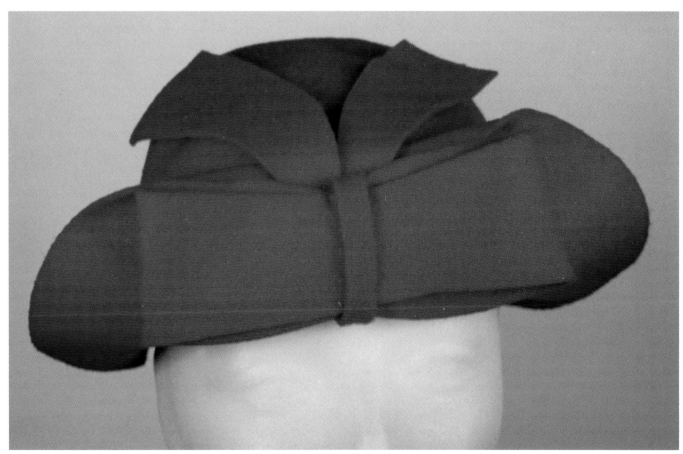

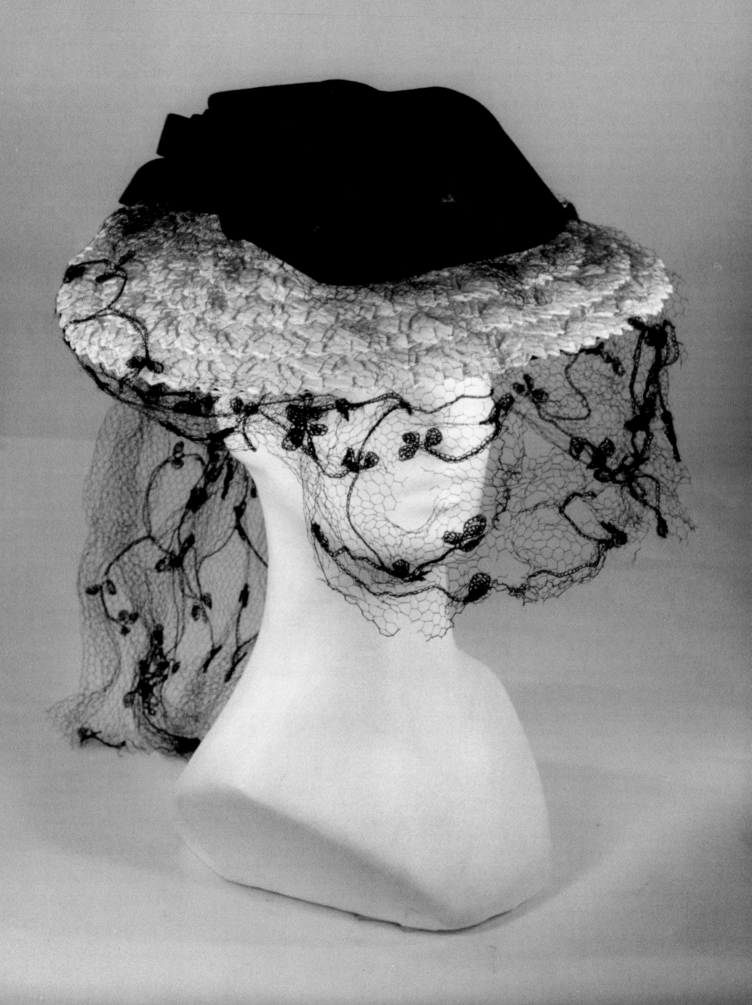

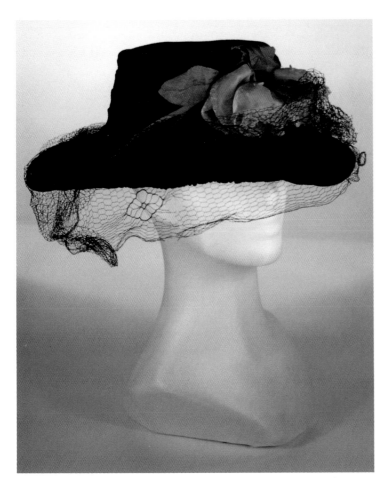

Ca. 1940 wide-brimmed silk hat, designed in a tricorne shape and decorated with mauve and tan silk flowers and an elaborately detailed black veil; lined with black silk.

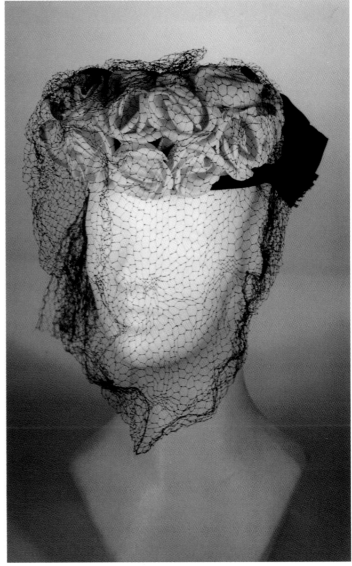

Ca. 1945 black velvet hat, trimmed with a cluster of ivory, cotton roses and a black veil.

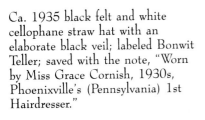

Ca. 1935 black felt and white cellophane straw hat with an elaborate black veil; labeled Bonwit Teller; saved with the note, "Worn by Miss Grace Cornish, 1930s, Phoenixville's (Pennsylvania) 1st Hairdresser."

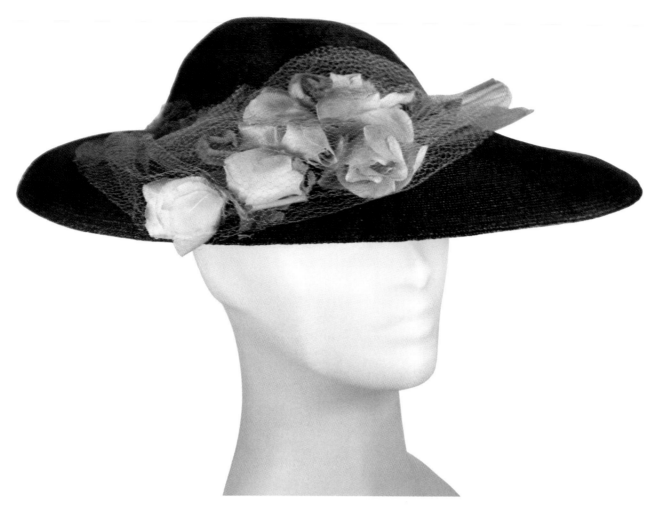

Ca. 1950 wide-brimmed, dyed black straw hat decorated with blue silk roses with cotton stems and an overlay of green net.

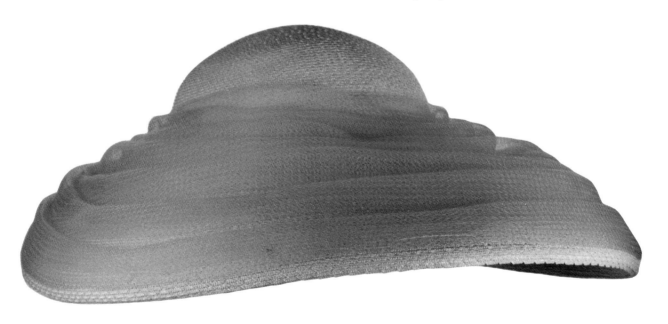

Ca. 1950 dyed-pink straw "picture hat," decorated with pink silk chiffon.

Ca. 1950 silk and velvet hat, designed as overlapping, hand painted "petals."

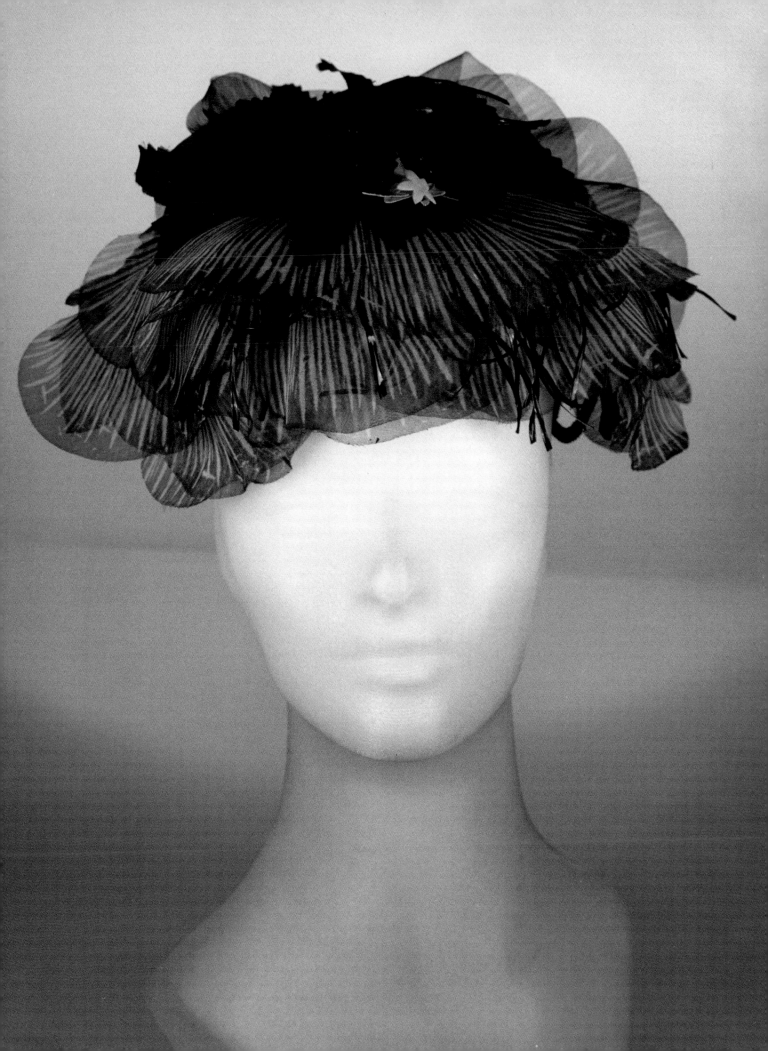

While *Vintage Style* attempts to showcase a number of wearable styles from 1920 to 1960, the most important goal here is to provide a survey designed to help collectors identify styles, trends, and dates of hats from 1876 to 1950. The illustrations presented were culled from thousands of sketches and photographs appearing in *The Millinery Trade Review* and its successor publication, *Hats*. This information was presented in the *Seventy-fifth Anniversary Issue of Hats*, published by the Millinery Trade Associates in 1951.

These illustrations become an invaluable dating tool for vintage hats, but millinery, as with the rest of fashion, is constantly being redesigned and reinterpreted. Even with the best of dating tools, dating hats is imprecise.

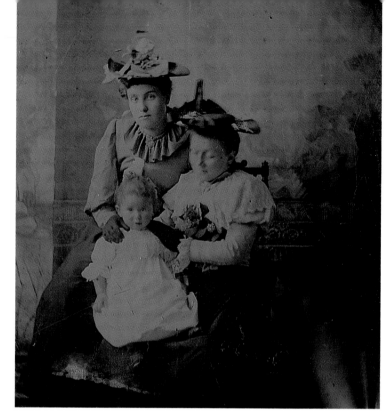

"The thing speaks for itself." *Photograph courtesy of David Sterner.*

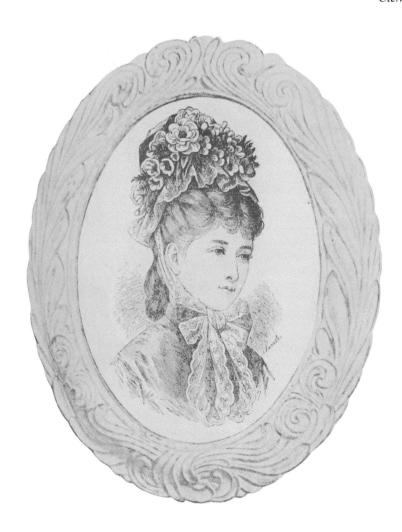

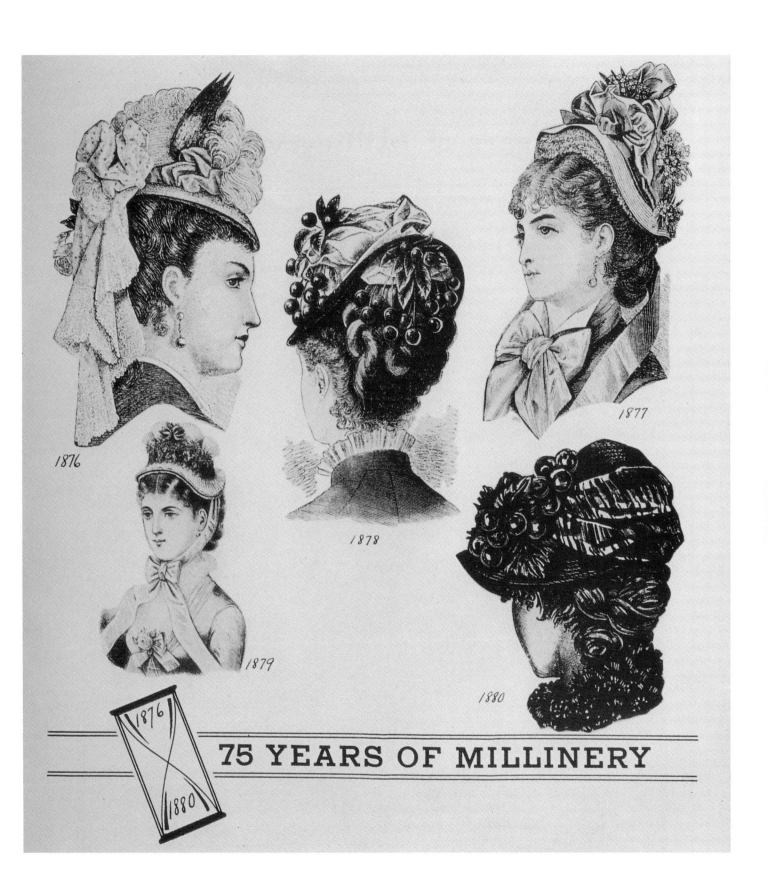

1876

1878

1877

1879

1880

1876
1880

75 YEARS OF MILLINERY

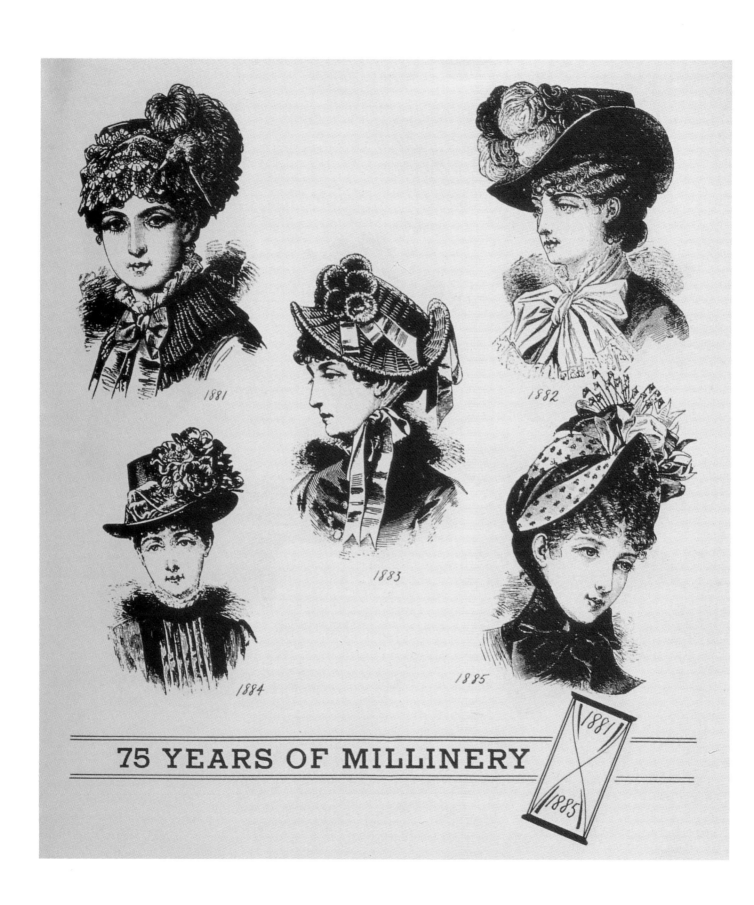

1881

1882

1883

1884

1885

75 YEARS OF MILLINERY

1881

1885

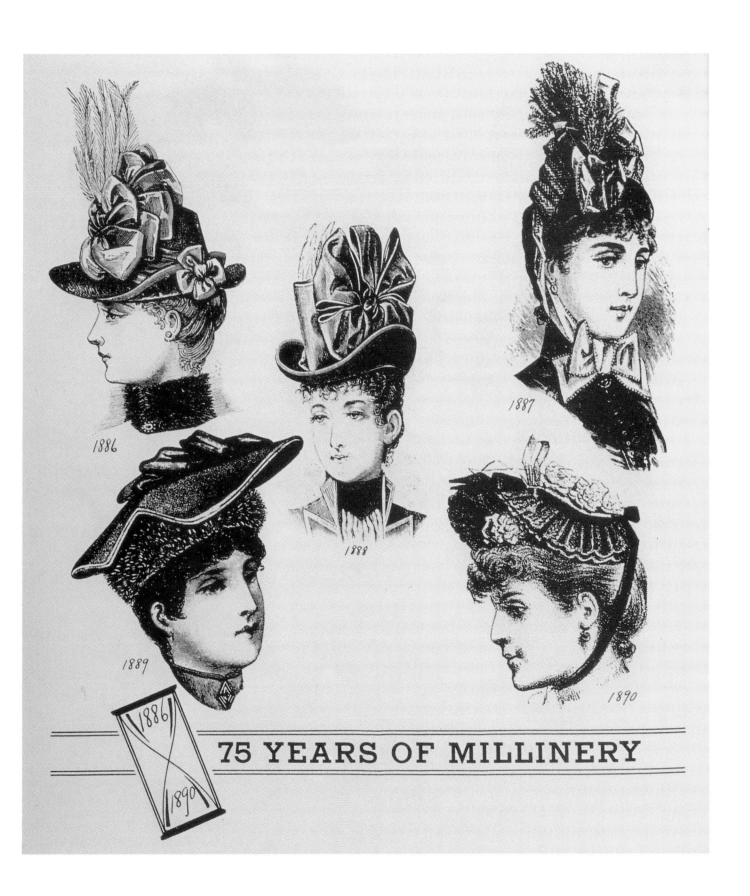

1886

1887

1888

1889

1890

1886
1890

75 YEARS OF MILLINERY

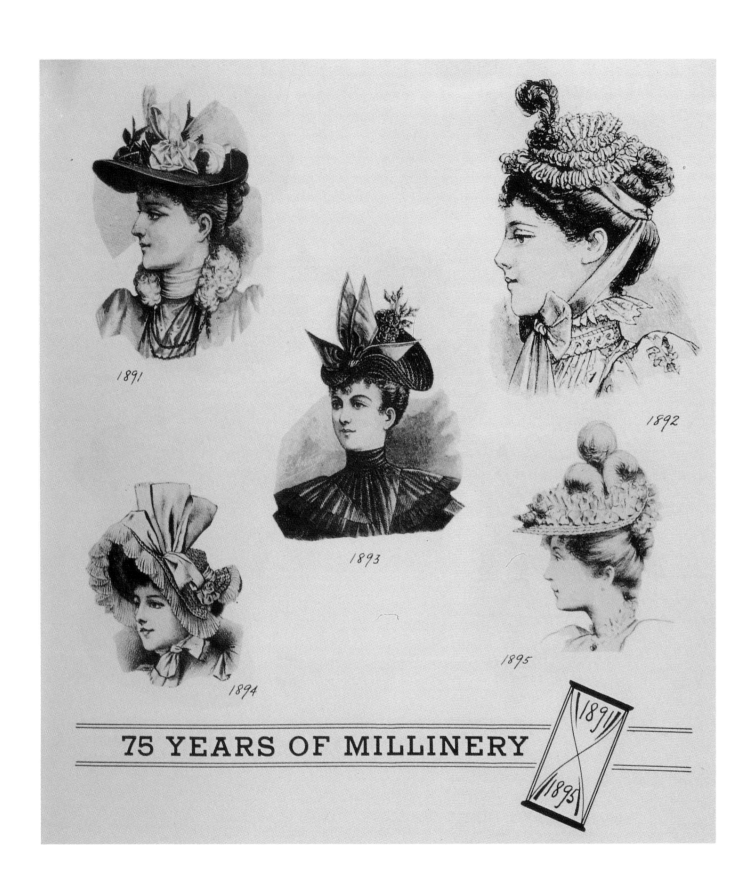

1891

1892

1893

1894

1895

75 YEARS OF MILLINERY

1891
1895

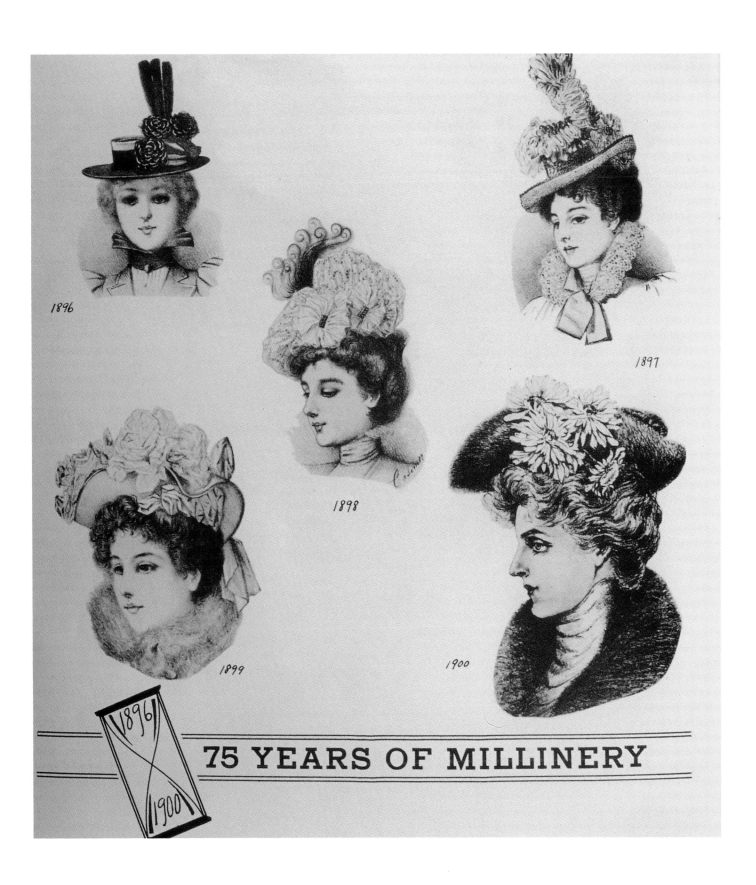

1896

1897

1898

1899

1900

1896
1900

75 YEARS OF MILLINERY

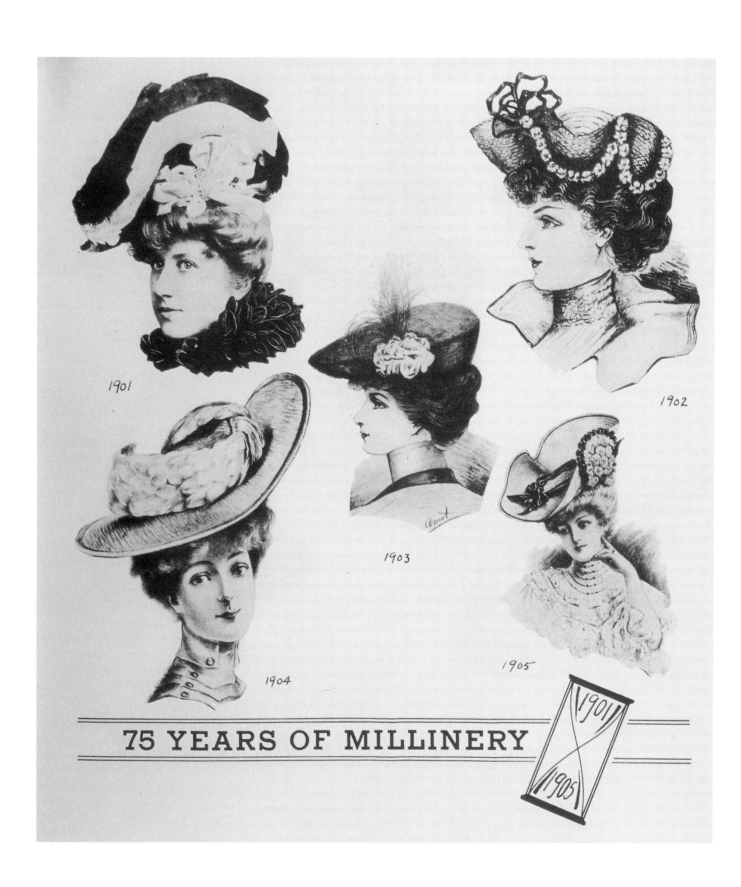

1901

1902

1903

1904

1905

75 YEARS OF MILLINERY

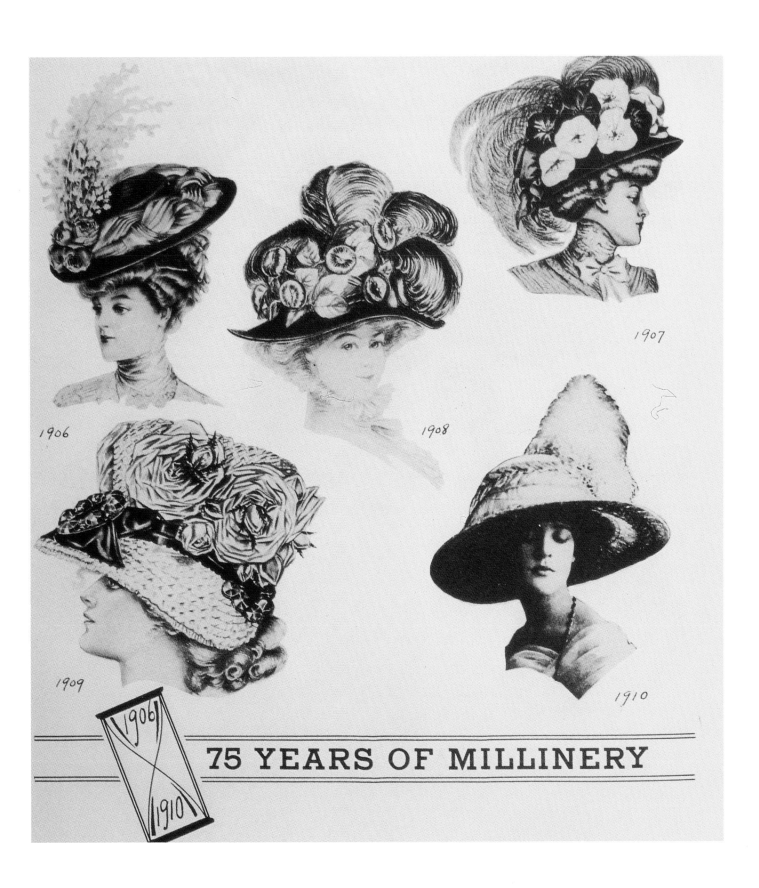

1906

1908

1907

1909

1910

1906
1910

75 YEARS OF MILLINERY

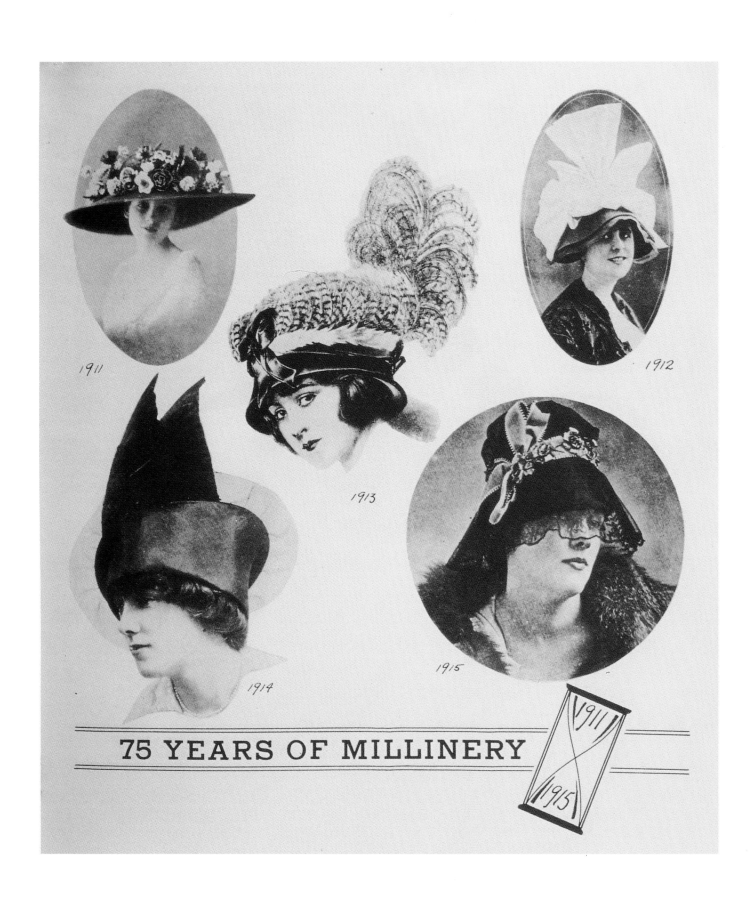

1911

1912

1913

1914

1915

75 YEARS OF MILLINERY

1911
1915

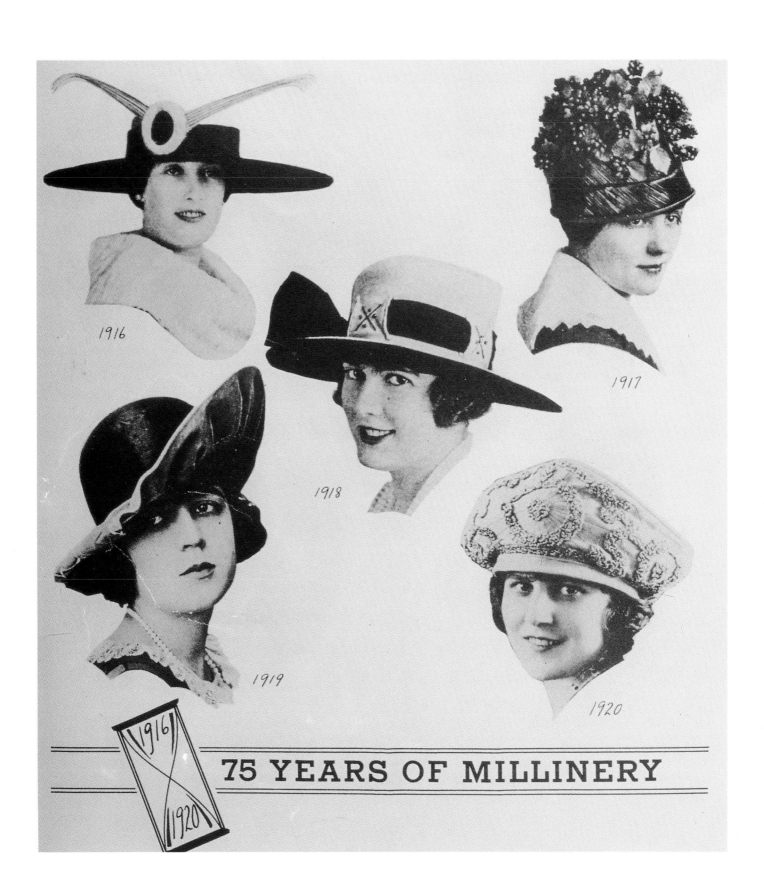

1916

1917

1918

1919

1920

1916
1920

75 YEARS OF MILLINERY

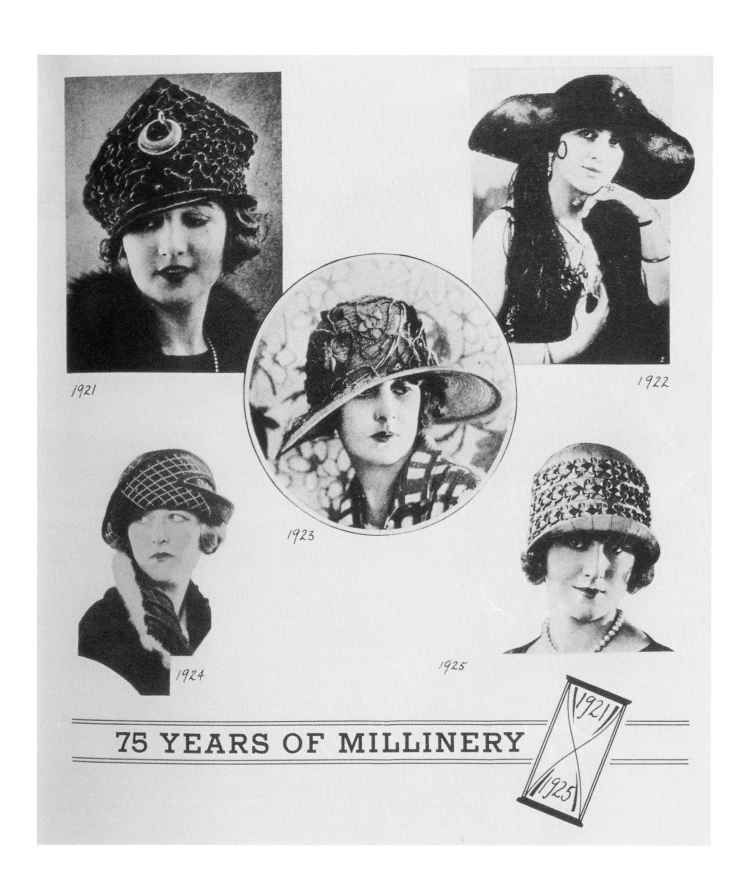

1921

1922

1923

1924

1925

75 YEARS OF MILLINERY

1921
1925

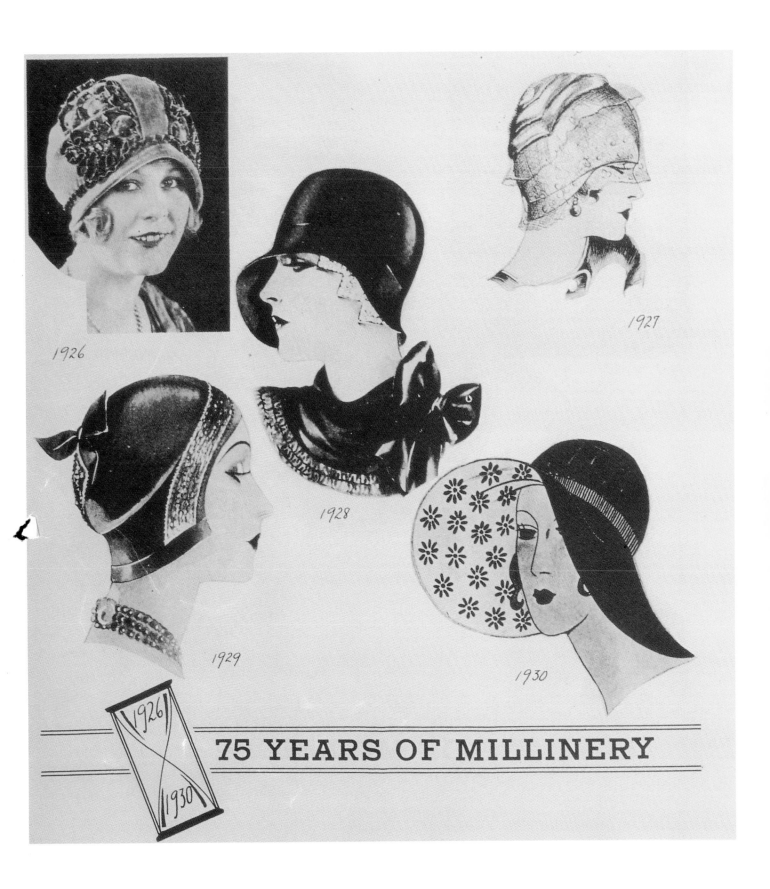

1926

1927

1928

1929

1930

75 YEARS OF MILLINERY

1926
1930

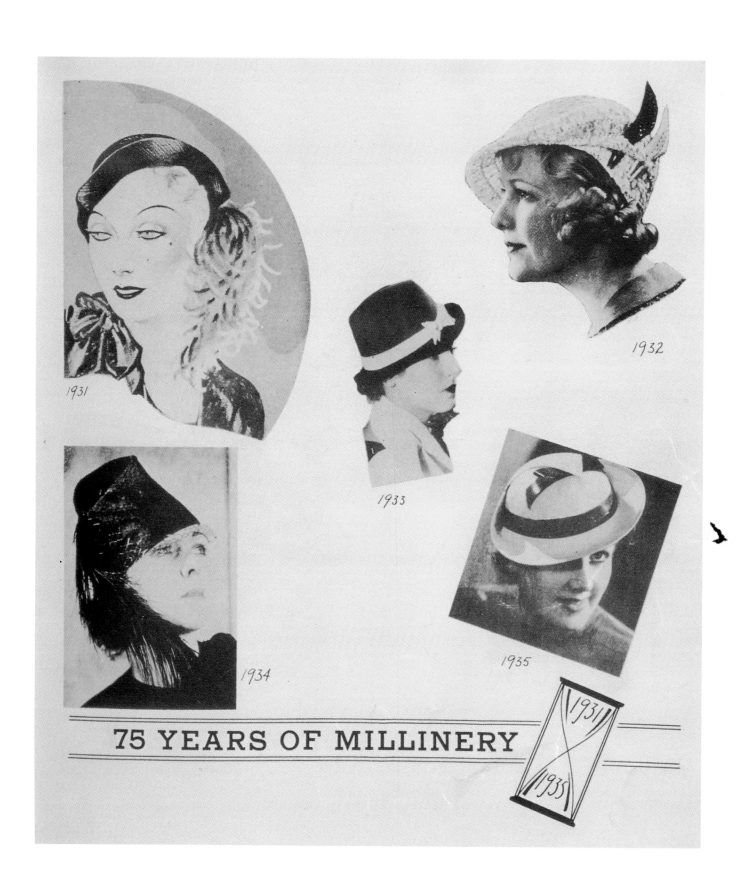

1931

1932

1933

1934

1935

75 YEARS OF MILLINERY

1931
1935

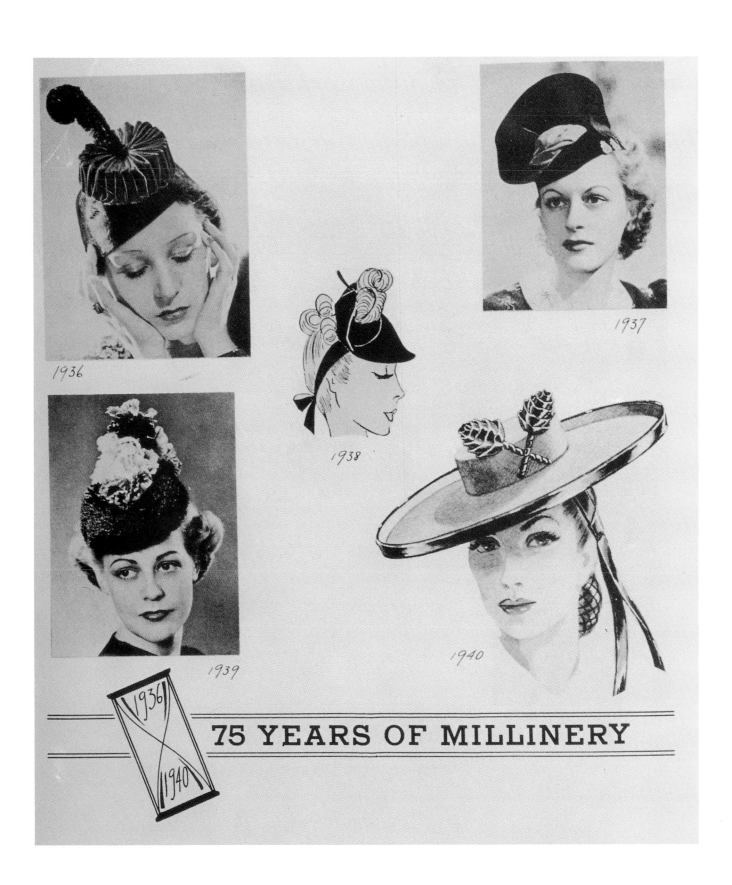

1936

1957

1938

1939

1940

75 YEARS OF MILLINERY

1936
1940

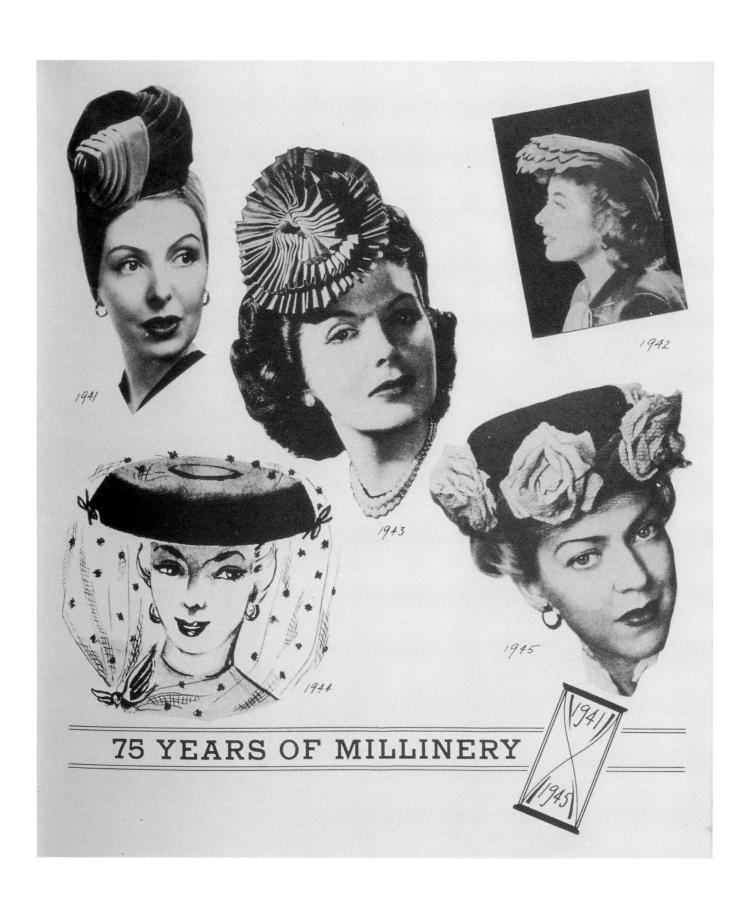

1941

1942

1943

1944

1945

75 YEARS OF MILLINERY

1941

1945

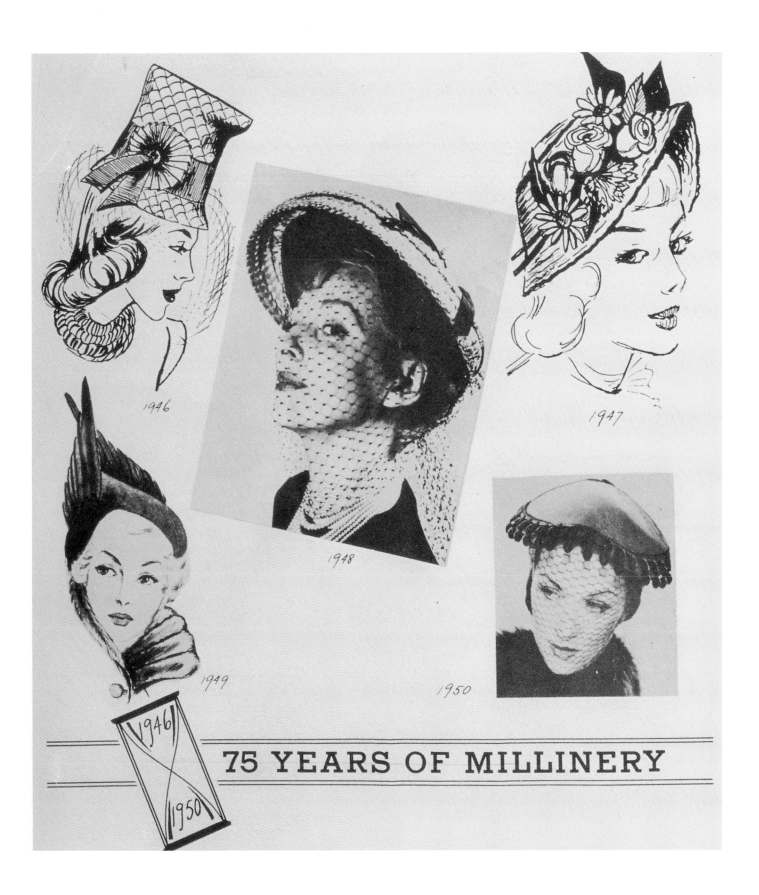

1946

1948

1947

1949

1950

1946
1950

75 YEARS OF MILLINERY

Glossary

Definitions are provided for terms used in the book which may not be clear from the context.

accordion pocketbook Bag made like an expandable file folder which is narrow at the top and pleated at the sides and bottom. Made with a handle and usually with a zipper compartment in the center.

Adrian, Gilbert American designer, 1903-1959. Born Gilbert Adrian Greenburgh in Naugatuck, Connecticut. Designed for Metro-Goldwyn-Mayer Studios from 1923 to 1939 for such stars as Joan Crawford, Greta Garbo, Norma Shearer, Katherine Hepburn, and Rosalind Russell. Opened retail business in Beverly Hills in 1941, for high priced "ready-to-wear" and couture; closed retail business in 1948, but continued in wholesale until 1953. Adrian retired to live in Brazil in 1952 with his wife, movie star Janet Gaynor, spending much of his time painting landscapes. He died in 1959.

aigrette Extremely long, delicate, white feather with a plume at the tip, from the egret, a long-legged wading bird which became almost extinct from the excesses of fashion.

alligator Leather from alligators with characteristic markings of blocks, rectangles, and circles with cross markings between. A law was passed in 1970 prohibiting its use in the United States; however, it has been relaxed somewhat since then.

ankle strap shoe A shoe, often a sandal, having a strap attached at the top of the heel which goes around the ankle.

aulmoniere A medieval pouch of silk or leather suspended from the girdle worn by nobles of the 13th century until the Reformation to carry alms.

baby Louis heel A low version of the **Louis** heel, a heel of medium height, curved sharply inward around sides and back, then flared slightly at base, similar to the heels worn in the Louis XV period.

Balenciaga, Cristobal Spanish-French couturier, 1895-1972. Born in Guetaria, Spain, son of a fishing-boat captain and a seamstress; after copying a Paris suit for a rich marquesa at age fourteen, he was encouraged to leave home to study fashion design. Eventually he supervised three of his own fashion houses called *Eisa*, in Madrid, San Sebastian, and Barcelona. In 1937 he opened his own business in Paris on Ave. Georges V, and was very successful. Balenciaga could design, cut, sew, and fit an entire garment, and was revered as the "Master" by his staff and peers. He created elegant clothes for royalty, film stars, and socialites, retiring in 1968. He came out of retirement to design the wedding dress for Carmencita de Martinez Bordiu in 1972, and died shortly after.

barrel pocketbook Handbag shaped like a stubby cylinder with a zipper closing and handles attached to the sides, like a small "barrel."

bias cut Manner of cutting diagonally across the grain of the fabric, resulting in a garment that closely follows the body's curves.

bolero jacket A rib-length jacket, open in front, with or without sleeves. Very popular during the 1950s, similar in style to jackets worn by bull fighters, these jackets first became popular at the end of the 19th century.

bouffant skirt Any full or gathered skirt.

box handbag A handbag with a rigid frame, similar to a small suitcase or lunch box.

bracelet handbag Type of handbag with one or two bracelets as handles.

Callot Soeurs (kal-o-sir) French couture house, 1895-1935. One of the great Paris dressmaking houses from 1916 to 1927. Firm founded in 1895 as a lace shop by three sisters, daughters of an antiques dealer. The eldest, Mme. Gerber, ran the business, and was an influence on one of their modellistes, Madeleine Vionnet. Famous for delicate lace blouses; gold and silver lame; Renaissance patterns; much chiffon, georgette, and organdy; rococo flower embroidery. Closed in 1937.

Chambre Syndicale de la Couture Parisienne An organization founded in 1868 by Parisian couturiers to regulate its members in regard to piracy of styles, dates of openings for collections, number of models presented, relations with the press, questions relating to law and taxes, and promotional activities.

Chambre Syndicale de la Mode An organization of milliners founded in Paris.

Chambre Syndicale des Paruriers An organization for accessories' houses, founded in Paris.

Chambre Syndicale du Prêt-à-Porter des Couturiers et Createurs de Mode An organization founded in Paris in 1975 to promote ready-to-wear and couture designers.

Chapman, Ceil American designer, 1912-. Born on Staten Island, New York, Ceil Chapman started her own "ready-to wear" business in 1940 (with first husband, Samuel Chapman); costumed the musical, *South Pacific,* and made clothes for Faye Emerson to wear on her television program. She specialized in cocktail dresses, rarely using printed fabrics, but relying for decoration on sequins, beading, and machine stitching.

chemise dress A dress fashionable after World War I that became the basic style of the 1920s. Made in a variety of styles and materials for day and evening wear.

chunky heeled shoe Shoes made in exaggeratedly heavy shapes with bulbous toes and massive heels, often with thick platform soles; a fad in late 1960s and early 1970s, and again in the late 1990s.

cloche hat A deep-crowned hat with very narrow brim fitting the head closely, concealing the hair, and worn pulled down to the eyebrows. Derived from the French word for "bell," the cloche was popular in the 1920s, 1960s, and again in the 1990s.

clutch handbag Frequently made in the envelope style, the clutch is a without a handle, but may have a strap on the back for carrying purposes. The "mini-clutch" is a tiny version of this bag, and may be elaborately beaded for evening wear.

couture A French term used throughout the fashion industry to describe the original styles, the ultimate in fine sewing and tailoring, the finest and most expensive fabrics.

crepe A wide variety of fabrics go under this name but usually have another name attached to define them further, such as "crepe de chine" (fine, lightweight silk fabric with a crepe texture). All fabrics are related as they have a slightly pebbly texture.

crinoline An open-weave cotton fabric which is heavily sized to be used for stiffening. A stiffened petticoat, worn to fill-out a skirt.

crocodile Thick skinned leather, from a large water reptile, characterized by black markings and a scaly, horny surface; very similar to alligator.

Daché, Lilly American designer, 1904-1989. Leading milliner in the United States from the late 1930s to late 1950s. Born in Beigles, France, Daché apprenticed at Reboux in Paris for four years, then came to New York in 1924. Worked as a milliner; sold hats at Macy's, opened her own shop where she molded hats on her customers and established her reputation. Bought her own building on East 56th Street in 1937, which was her home, workroom, and showroom. By 1949 she was designing clothes to go with her hats, gloves, hosiery, lingerie, wallets, and jewelry. In 1954 she added perfume and cosmetics. Closed business in 1969. Wrote two books about fashion, *Talking Through My Hats* and *Glamour Unlimited*.

designer Person involved in creating original clothing and accessories. Some designers own their own businesses, others are employed by manufacturers to create collections of merchandise in couture, "ready-to wear," lingerie, millinery, footwear, accessories, and jewelry.

Dior, Christian, French couturier, 1905-1957. Born in Granville, France (Normandy); son of a rich industrialist. Operated an art gallery from 1930 to 1934; sketched hat designs for Agnès; designed for Piguet in 1938, and for Lucien Lelong in 1941. Opened own house on Ave. Montaign in 1947; launched the revolutionary "new look"--a feminine silhouette, yards of material in an almost ankle-length skirt, with a tiny waist, snug bodice, sloping shoulders, and padded hips. In next ten years, he invented his own inner constructions to shape a dress into and "H," "A," or "Y" line. From 1948 to 1951 he added perfumes, scarfs, hosiery, furs, gloves, men's neckties, and a less expensive, young line, "Miss Dior," which became an international merchandising operation. After his death, house continued under the leadership of his assistant, Yves Saint Laurent, from 1957 to 1960, and since then with Marc Bohan.

dirndl skirt A skirt which is cut full and gathered into a band at the waist, popular in the 1940s and 1950s.

Duskin, Nan A Russian immigrant who worked briefly for the Blum Store in Philadelphia, and then opened her own retail store for women's clothing and accessories at 1729 Walnut Street, Philadelphia, Pennsylvania. She was known for her excellent taste, and bought only the best examples of the work of the greatest designers in the world, and exceptionally interesting or special "ready-to-wear" items. She had a shrewd head for business and hired only the most capable workers, including her buyer, Carol Greeny, a former model who worked at the store for many years. Nan Duskin let it be known that she was interested in hiring only "ladies, not salesladies" to work for her. Many of the workers were former Nan Duskin models. She sold the business in the late 1970s. It is said that at the exact hour of her death, the lights in the store dimmed and went out. After Nan Duskin, the business had two owners, before it closed in November, 1994.

Eisenberg & Sons Originals A wholesale fashion company founded in Chicago in 1914 by Jonas Eisenberg. In the 1930s the company specialized in little black crepe dinner dresses and gowns, decorated with costume jewelry, crystal buttons, embroidered and jeweled belts, collars, and cuffs. The story goes that customers were taking the costume jewelry off clothing in the Chicago store, and that this is why the company began making the jewelry to be sold separately. The crystal used in the costume jewelry was imported from D. Swarovski & Company in Austria. Eisenberg & Sons Originals stopped making clothes in the late 1950s.

Empress Eugénie hat A small hat popular in the 1930s, pitched forward to one side of the face; style is based on a hat worn by Empress Eugénie, the wife of Napoleon III (1852-1870).

ensemble The entire costume, including accessories, worn at one time.

Fath, Jacques French couturier, 1912-1954. Great-grandson of designer Empress Eugénie, grandson of a painter, son of Alsatian businessman. Opened his own fashion house in 1937, which he kept open during the war, and for the next seventeen years he was very successful, designing elegant, flattering, feminine clothing. He also had a boutique for perfume, stockings, scarfs, and millinery. Married to actress, Genevieve Boucher de la Bruyere. Died of leukemia at age forty-two in 1954. His business was carried on by his wife until 1957.

filet lace Hand knotted lace with square holes, frequently filled-in with colored yarns in a darning stitch.

fittings The trade term for the dressmaker's or tailor's session with the customer for altering the garment to fit the customer.

Fogarty, Anne American designer, 1919-1981. Designed junior-size dresses between 1948 and 1957 for Youth Guild and Margot, Inc., at Saks Fifth Avenue from 1957 to 1962; established Anne Fogarty, Inc. in 1962. Completed a spring/summer collection of dresses and sportswear shortly before her death in 1981. Designs included lingerie, jewelry, shoes, hats, coats, and suits.

fold-over clutch pocketbook Envelope style handbag which may be open at the top or have a zippered closing. Bag is folded over double and carried in the hand or under the arm.

Fortuny, Mariano Mariano Fortuny y Madrazo, Italian designer, 1871-1949. Born in Venice, he was an innovator, inventor, photographer, stage designer, and textile and dress designer. He is famous for his long, slender, mushroom-pleated silk teagowns, slipped over the head and tied at the waist by a thin silk cord. His most famous design, the Delphos gown, appeared in 1907. His unique pleating technique was first shown in Paris in 1910, and the method he used remains a mystery today. His clothes, which were considered classic throughout the 1930s, are now rare collector's items!

frog An ornamental fastener, made of braid or cording, used for closing garments; introduced in the West from China in the last quarter of the 18th century.

gabardine Durable, closely woven fabric with noticeable ridges caused by the warp-faced twill weave. May be made of cotton, wool, or rayon.

Galanos, James American designer, 1929-. Born in Philadelphia of Greek immigrants. Studied fashion in New York; worked at Robert Piguet in Paris from 1947 to 1948, and then returned to New York. Started his own business in Los Angeles in 1951, and his first show in New York in 1952 launched him on a spectacular career; in five years he received the Coty Award and was elected into the Hall of Fame. Known for luxurious day and evening ensembles; dresses many socialites and movie stars, including Nancy Reagan for the 1981 and 1985 Presidential Inaugural Balls. Lives in California, but shows only in New York.

Harlow pump Sabot-strap pump with a high, chunky heel popular in the early 1970s, named after shoes worn by Jean Harlow, a Hollywood actress of the 1920s and 1930s.

high top shoes A lace-up or button-up over the ankle, close-fitting boot, popular from 1890 to 1915, and later in many rural areas. The style became popular again in the 1990s.

International Ladies' Garment Workers' Union, The A semi-industrial union of United States and Canadian needle-trades workers, founded in 1900. A very strong union for many years, it has fewer members, and is less influential today.

Irene American designer, 1907-1962. Irene Lentz used her first name professionally. She began designing in her own boutique on the campus of the University of Southern California, Los Angeles, in the 1930s. She ran a boutique in Hollywood, and became the head of the custom department at Bullocks-Wilshire in Los Angeles, where many of her clients were film stars. When Adrian left Metro-Goldwyn-Mayer in 1942, Irene took over as head costumer, a job she kept until 1949. In 1947 she established a "ready-to-wear" business, specializing in tailored garments for day wear, and dramatic evening gowns.

L85 The government order during World War II which regulated the hem measurement of a skirt to 72" around and the trimming material in each dress to half a yard.

lapel The turned-back front section of a blouse, jacket, coat or shirt where it joins the collar. Each side folds back to form lapels, which are cut in different shapes.

l'Escole de la Chambre Syndicale de la Couture A school for couturiers founded in Paris in 1930.

Lilli Ann of San Francisco Company headed by Adolph Schumann, founded in early 1940s, and was very productive, manufacturing beautifully tailored suits and "swing" coats. Known for great detailing, and the 1940s silhouette.

Mary Jane shoes A low-heeled slipper made of patent leather with a blunt toe and a single strap over the instep, buttoned or buckled at the center or side. A trademark shoe for children, popular since the early 20th century. In the 1980s a flattie in a pump style with a buckled strap coming high over the instep. Named for the shoes worn by the character Mary Jane in the comic strip, Buster Brown, drawn by R. F. Outcault in the early 1900s.

McCardell, Claire American designer, 1906-1958. Studied at Parsons School in New York and in Paris. Worked for Robert Turk, Inc. as an assistant designer in 1929, worked at Townley Frocks, Inc., and remained as designer - partner until her death at age fifty-two. Credited with originating the American look.

mechlin lace Fragile bobbin lace with ornamental designs outlined with shiny cordonnets and placed on hexagonal net ground. Derived from the city of Mechlin, Belgium, where it was made.

mesh handbag Tiny links of metal joined to make a flexible bag, popular in the early 1900s in a small size, often with sterling silver frames. In the 1940s, mesh handbags were made with larger white enameled links and white plastic frames.

millinery Women's head coverings, specifically hats, bonnets, caps, hoods, and veils.

minaudiere A small, rigid metal evening bag used to hold cosmetics made in oval, oblong or square shapes. Carried in the hand or by a short chain. Decorated with engraved designs or set with jewels.

Molyneux, Edward French couturier, 1891-1974. Born in Ireland, started working at age seventeen in London, Chicago, and New York as a designer with Lucile. He was a captain in the British Army during World War I, where he lost an eye. Opened own house in Paris in 1919, on rue Royale, and designed elegant clothing for such celebrities as Lynn Fontanne, Princess Marina, and the Duchess of Windsor. Worked for national defense, establishing international canteen during World War II, and returned to Paris house in 1949, adding furs, lingerie, millinery, and perfumes. One of the original members of the Incorporated Society of London Fashion Designers in 1942. Turned over Paris house to Jacques Griffe in 1950, and retired to Jamaica, West Indies. He came out of retirement to bring a "ready-to wear" collection to the United States in 1965, but the venture was unsuccessful.

needlepoint Wool embroidery worked all over open canvas with yarn in a variety of tapestry stitches either horizontally across the rows or diagonally, making it double-faced.

Norell, Norman American designer, 1900-1972. Born Norman Levinson in Noblesville, Indiana, son of haberdashery store owner in Indianapolis. Came to New York in 1919 to study at Parson's School of Design. Started with theatrical and movie designing for Paramount Pictures and Brooks Costume Company. In 1924 worked for Charles Armour, then for Hattie Carnegie from 1928 to 1940. Partnership in the firm Traina-Norell followed in 1941. After death of Traina in 1960, formed own company, Norman Norell, Inc. Rated as top American designer on Seventh Avenue, "Dean of the fashion industry," "the American Balenciaga." First designer elected to Hall of Fame by Coty Award judges in 1958. He suffered a stroke on the eve of his retrospective show at the Metropolitan Museum of Art, October 15, 1972, and died ten days later. The firm continued for a short time after his death under Gustave Tassel.

petal sleeves A short sleeve, curved at the hem, and overlapping to give a petal-shaped effect in front.

petit point Canvas embroidery worked from right to left, working over single threads through large meshes.

picture hat A hat with a large brim framing the face, frequently made of straw.

platform pump A shoe with a thick mid-sole, usually made of cork and covered so that the wearer appears taller. Popular for women in the 1940s, and revived by Paris designer, Yves Saint Laurent in the 1960s. Worn by men in the 1970s.

Poiret, Paul French designer, 1880-1944. Labeled King of Fashion from 1904 to 1924. Born in Paris, son of a cloth merchant; began by dressing wooden dolls; sold sketches to couturiers. First employed by Doucet in 1896, where he developed an interest in theatrical costuming. He worked for a short period for the House of Worth, then opened his own fashion house in 1904. He became known as a "tyrant over women," who imposed his original ideas and strident colors; banned the corset, and shackled legs with the harem and hobble skirts. He spent a fortune on costume balls and decorations of his home, and refused to change his "exotic image" in fashion, and, as a result, faded from the fashion scene. He died in Paris in 1944 after years of poverty and illness.

poodle cloth A knitted or woven fabric, characterized by small curls all over the surface, resembling the coat of a poodle dog.

poodle skirt A circular skirt, usually made of felt, which was popular during the mid- 1950s, and had a poodle dog appliqued on it, sometimes wearing a collar and leash. Such designs were often made of poodle cloth or felt of another color.

pouch handbag A basic style originally made of soft, shirred leather or fabric, with a drawstring closing. Now also made with a frame and handles.

prêt-à-porter A French term which translates as "ready to be carried," or clothes that are not custom made.

princess style dress A basic cut for women's clothing, characterized by continuous vertical panels, shaped to the body through the torso, without a waistline seam. Used in dresses, coats, and slips from 1860 on, and was especially popular in the late 1940s and early 1950s.

prom gown Term to describe semi-formal or formal gown worn to a formal dance or "prom" (short for "promenade"), usually held in April or May of the junior and senior years of high school. In the 1950s such gowns were often made of layers of net, tulle, silk chiffon, or nylon, in white or pastel shades, and many of these gowns were strapless.

Quant, Mary British designer, 1934-. Credited with starting the Chelsea or Mod Look in the mid-1950s, making London the most influential fashion center at that time. She was a pioneer of the body stocking, hot pants, and the layered look in dressing. At the age of twenty-three she had two shops, selling her own idea of spirited, unconventional clothes. By 1967, she had started the mini-skirt revolution. Married to Alexander Plunkett-Greene, her partner from the beginning.

ready-to-wear clothes Garments that are available in various sizes, and are "ready to be carried," as opposed to couture and custom made garments, which require individual fitting.

reticule Woman's small purse which may be made of satin, mesh, leather, and other materials. It took many shapes, including envelope, urn, circle, basket, and shell. Used from the late 19th to early 20th centuries. Also called "indispensible" and "ballantine."

Rouff, Maggy French couturier, 1897-1971, Although Maggy Rouff planned to be a surgeon, she decided on couture in 1918 and learned to cut and sew. Started own business in 1929 and for twenty-five years was among the leaders of Paris fashion. Work was known for its refined, feminine elegance. Retired in 1948.

Scaasi, Arnold American designer, 1930-. Born Arnold Isaacs in Montreal, Canada, he studied design in Canada and Paris before working as an apprentice at the house of Paquin. He moved to New York in 1951, and worked for just over two years with Charles James. When he began working on his own, he reversed the letters of his last name.

His early speciality was evening gowns, with matching coats. He also pioneered the knee-baring formal evening dress. In the mid-1960s he began custom designing again, and in the 1970s was known as New York's "only couturier," making clothes for a small group of private clients.

Schiaparelli, Elsa French couturiere, 1890-1973. Born in Rome, one of the most creative, unconventional couturieres of the 1930s and 1940s; an innovator whose clothes were startling conversation pieces. First designed dressmaker sweaters with designs knit in, such as a white collar and bow-tie on black. By 1929 had her own business, *Pour le Sport*, in rue de la Paix and first boutique at 4 Place Vendome in 1935. Great success with avant-garde sweaters with tattoo or skeleton motifs; hot pink color, "Shocking" perfume (which had an hourglass-torso bottle). Known for designing the first evening dress with its own jacket, trouser skirts for all occasions, use of zippers, padlocks and dog lease fastenings, doll hats (some shaped like lamb chops or pink-heeled shoes), and flying and golf suits. Traveled extensively and had close friendships with a number of artists, including Dali and Man Ray. Published her autobiography, *Shocking Life*, in 1954. Remained a consultant for companies licensed to produce merchandise under her name, but closed her business in 1954. After retirement, lived in Tunisia and Paris, where she died in 1973.

sizing A term to describe the cutting of garments in various sizes to fit a variety of body types.

snakeskin Diamond-patterned leather with overlapping scales processed from the skin of a number of species of snakes, including diamond-backed rattlesnake, python, cobra, and boa.

soutache Narrow, flat decorative braid of mohair, silk, or rayon. Used for borders and for all over ornamental patterns. Also called Russian braid.

tote handbag A utility bag which is large enough to carry small packages. It was copied from the shape of a common paper shopping bag.

Trigere, Pauline American designer, 1912-. Born in Paris and came to New York in 1937, where she worked for Travis Banton for Hattie Carnegie. Started New York business in 1941 with her brother, Robert. Her son, Jean-Pierre Radley is president of Trigere, Inc. Specializes in coats, suits, capes, dresses and accessories in unusual tweeds and prints, with intricate cut to flatter mature figures. Licenses include scarfs, jewelry, furs, men's neckties, sunglasses, bedroom fashions, paperworks, servingware, and fragrance. Her trademark is the "turtle." Design students who have met and talked with Trigere describe her as an exceptional designer, who is very kind, encouraging, and willing to share her ideas with them.

Vionnet, Madeleine French couturiere, 1876-1975. Considered to be one of the three greatest fashion designers of the 20th century, ranking with Chanel and Balenciaga in contributions and lasting influence. She has been called the greatest technician of modern couture for her innovation of the bias cut and freeing of the body from corsetry and whalebone necklines. Born in Aubervilliers, France, she began dressmaking at an early age, training in London and in Paris with Mme. Gerber at Callot, and in 1907 with Doucet. She opened her own house in 1912, closing down during World War I, and opening again in 1922 on the avenue Montaigne. She closed finally before World War II, in 1940. A Vionnet dress was noted for classical drapery, for wide-open necklines, easy over-the-head entry, suppression of hooks and eyes, cowl or halter necks, handkerchief-point hem; faggoted seams; Art Deco embroideries, difficult to copy. She is known for having draped and cut her designs on small wooden mannequins. She died on March 2, 1975 in Paris.

Woolworth shoe Made of cotton canvas in a sandal style, in shades of red, navy, paisley, black, or white, this shoe has been sold at Woolworth stores for fifty years. Also called the "landlady shoe."

Worth, Charles Frederick French couturier, 1826-1895. Born in Bourne, Lincolnshire, England. Famous during the 19th century as the dressmaker for Empress Eugénie and the court of France's Second Empire. Considered to be the founder of the industry of *haute couture*. After serving an apprenticeship in London drapery establishments, he came to Paris in 1845, at age twenty, to work for a dealer in fabrics, shawls, and mantels. In 1858, he opened his own house on rue de la Paix, called Worth et Bobergh, which was closed during the Franco-Prussian War (1870-1871) and opened as Maison Worth in 1874, with his sons Jean Phillipe and Gaston. For fifty years the house was a fashion leader without rivals, dressing ladies of the courts and society all over Europe and America. Famous for the princess-cut dress, the collapsible steel framework for crinolines, and later the elimination of crinolines (1867), gowns made of interchangeable parts (various combinations of bodice, sleeve, and skirt with infinite variety of trimming). Worth was the innovator in the presentation of gowns on live mannequins, and the first to sell models to be copied in the United States and England. Opened house in London and introduced Parfums Worth in 1900, and "Je Reviens," the best known fragrance. After his death in 1895, the house continued under his sons and grandsons. It was sold to Paquin in 1954.

Bibliography

Fairchild's Dictionary of Fashion, 2nd Edition. Edited by Charlotte Mankey Calasibetta. New York: Fairchild Publications, 1988.

Hartley, E. F. *Clues to American Dress*. Washington, D. C.: Starrhill Press, 1994.

Hats: Seventy-fifth Anniversary Issue, published by the Millinery Trade Associates in 1951.

Milbank, Caroline Rennolds. *New York Fashion: The Evolution of American Style*. New York: Harry N. Abrams, Inc., Publishers, Paper bound Edition, 1996.

Wanamaker Diary, The. Philadelphia, John Wanamaker, 1933.

Price Reference

Regional differences, trends, and selling venue dramatically affect the prices of vintage clothing and accessories. Highest prices are always paid for items in excellent condition. Couture clothing is a specialized interest area, and the prices tend to be as unpredictable as the stock market. Prices given are for items in *excellent* condition. Similar items in *poor* condition may have little or no value. Prices are unavailable for items pictured which are part of institutional or individual costume collections.

NPA= No Price Available

Page	$
Half title and title page	115-125
Page 6	125-130
Page 10 on model	300-350
Page 11	115-125
Page 12	1500-2000
Page 14	400-425
Page 15	200-225
Pages 16-17	1000-1250
Pages 18-19	NPA
Pages 20-21	NPA
Pages 22-23	NPA
Page 24	525-600
Page 25	225-275
Pages 26-27	NPA
Page 28	NPA
Page 29 left	300-325
right	125-150
Page 30 left	185-200
right	200-225
Page 31 on model	195-225
Page 32	175-200
Page 33 left	75-95
right	150-175
Page 34 left	175-200
right	NPA

Page	$
Page 35 left	185-225
right	250-275
Page 36 on model	45-65
Page 37	950-975
Page 38 left	375-425
bottom right	150-175
Page 39 left	NPA
right	65-85
Page 40 left	175-225
right	150-175
Page 41 bottom left	50-60
right	50-60
Page 42 left	95-110
right	95-110
Page 43 left	85-95
right	95-110
Page 44	NPA
Page 45	1000-1250
Page 46	85-110
Page 47	85-110
Page 48 left	NPA
right	150-185
Page 49	550-600
Page 50 left	325-350
right	300-325
Page 51	350-400
Page 52 left	85-95
bottom right	45-65

Index

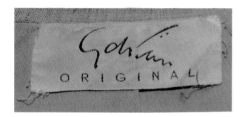
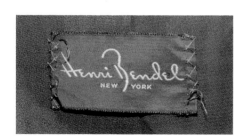
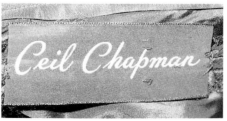
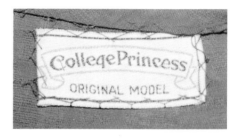
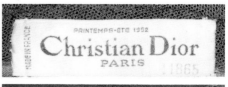
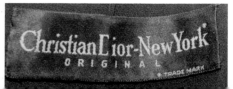

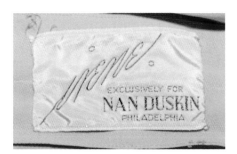

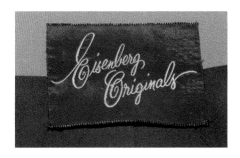

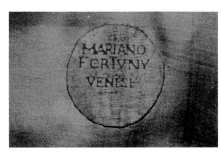

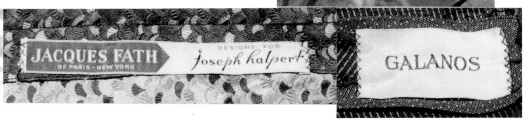

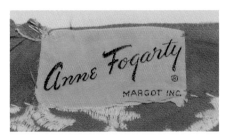

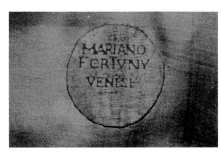

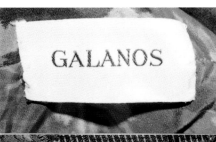

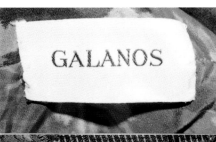

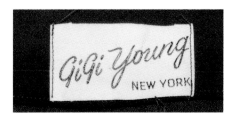

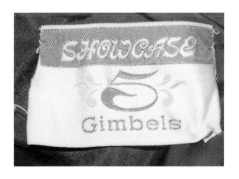

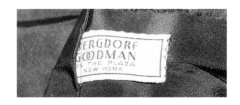

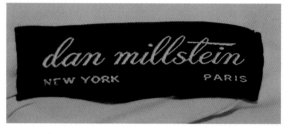

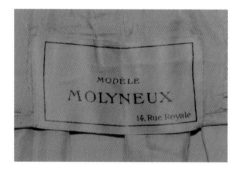

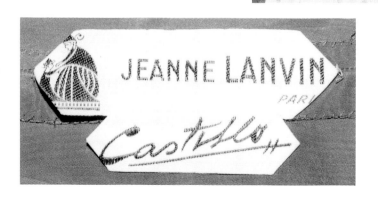

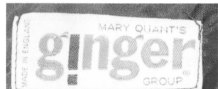

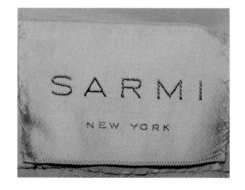

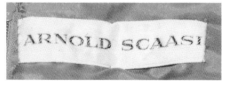

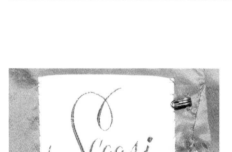

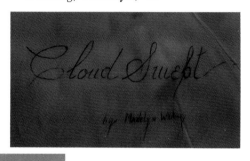

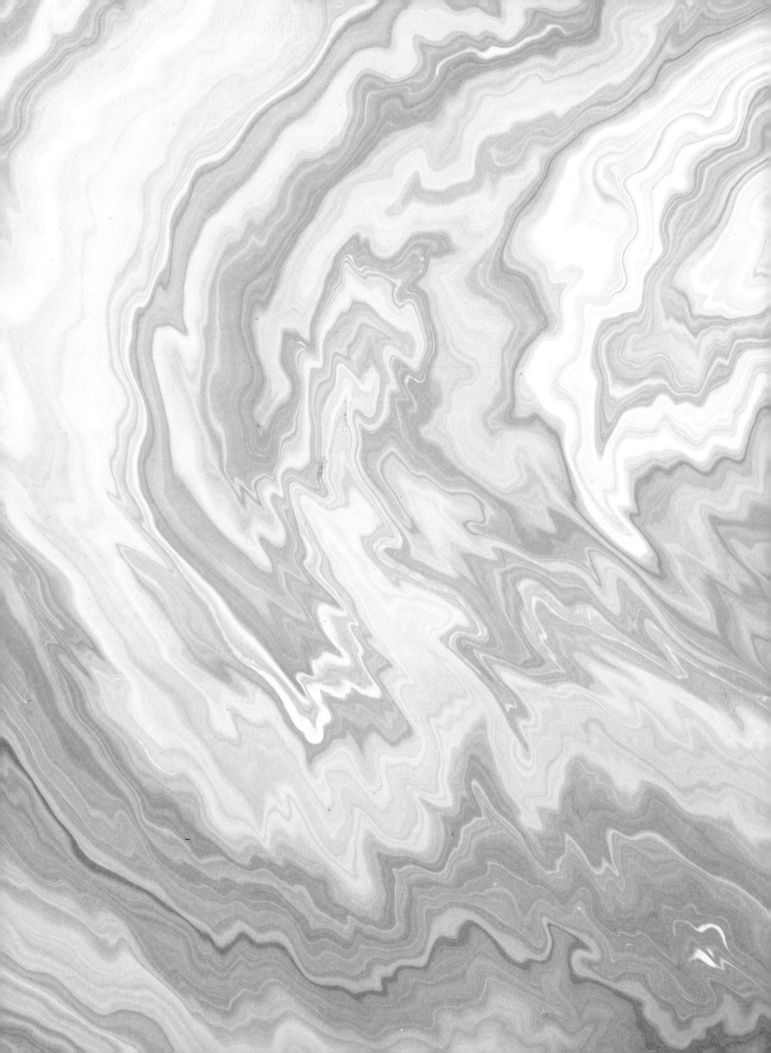